Gary W. Elmer, PhD
Lynne V. McFarland, PhD
Marc McFarland

The Power of Probiotics
Improving Your Health
with Beneficial Microbes

The Power of Probiotics
Improving Your Health with Beneficial Microbes

THE HAWORTH PRESS®
Haworth Series in Integrative Healing
Ethan Russo
Editor

The Last Sorcerer: Echoes of the Rainforest by Ethan Russo

Professionalism and Ethics in Complementary and Alternative Medicine by John Crellin and Fernando Ania

Cannabis and Cannabinoids: Pharmacology, Toxicology, and Therapeutic Potential by Franjo Grotenhermen and Ethan Russo

Modern Psychology and Ancient Wisdom: Psychological Healing Practices from the World's Religious Traditions edited by Sharon G. Mijares

Complementary and Alternative Medicine: Clinic Design by Robert A. Roush

Herbal Voices: American Herbalism Through the Words of American Herbalists by Anne K. Dougherty

The Healing Power of Chinese Herbs and Medicinal Recipes by Joseph P. Hou and Youyu Jin

Alternative Therapies in the Treatment of Brain Injury and Neurobehavioral Disorders: A Practical Guide edited by Gregory J. Murrey

Handbook of Cannabis Therapeutics: From Bench to Bedside edited by Ethan B. Russo and Franjo Grotenhermen

The Power of Probiotics: Improving Your Health with Beneficial Microbes by Gary W. Elmer, Lynne V. McFarland, and Marc McFarland

The Power of Probiotics
Improving Your Health with Beneficial Microbes

Gary W. Elmer, PhD
Lynne V. McFarland, PhD
Marc McFarland

The Haworth Press
New York • London • Oxford

For more information on this book or to order, visit
http://www.haworthpress.com/store/product.asp?sku=5597

or call 1-800-HAWORTH (800-429-6784) in the United States and Canada
or (607) 722-5857 outside the United States and Canada

or contact orders@HaworthPress.com

PUBLISHER'S NOTE
The development, preparation, and publication of this work has been undertaken with great care. However, the Publisher, employees, editors, and agents of The Haworth Press are not responsible for any errors contained herein or for consequences that may ensue from use of materials or information contained in this work. The Haworth Press is committed to the dissemination of ideas and information according to the highest standards of intellectual freedom and the free exchange of ideas. Statements made and opinions expressed in this publication do not necessarily reflect the views of the Publisher, Directors, management, or staff of The Haworth Press, Inc., or an endorsement by them.

This book has been published solely for educational purposes and is not intended to substitute for the medical advice of a treating physician. Medicine is an ever-changing science. As new research and clinical experience broaden our knowledge, changes in treatment may be required. While many potential treatment options are made herein, some or all of the options may not be applicable to a particular individual. Therefore, the author, editor, and publisher do not accept responsibility in the event of negative consequences incurred as a result of the information presented in this book. We do not claim that this information is necessarily accurate by the rigid scientific and regulatory standards applied for medical treatment. **No warranty, expressed or implied, is furnished with respect to the material contained in this book. The reader is urged to consult with his/her personal physician with respect to the treatment of any medical condition.**

The views expressed in this book are those of the authors and do not necessarily reflect the position or policy of the Department of Veterans Affairs.

Cover design by Jennifer M. Gaska.

Library of Congress Cataloging-in-Publication Data

Elmer, Gary.
    The power of probiotics : improving your health with beneficial microbes / Gary Wells Elmer, Lynne V. McFarland, Marc McFarland.
       p. cm.
    Includes index and bibliographical references.
    ISBN-13: 978-0-7890-2900-3 (case 13 : alk. paper)
    ISBN-10: 0-7890-2900-6 (case 10 : alk. paper)
    ISBN-13: 978-0-7890-2901-0 (soft 13 : alk. paper)
    ISBN-10: 0-7890-2901-4 (soft 10 : alk. paper)
    1. Probiotics—Therapeutic use. I. McFarland, Lynne V. II. McFarland, Marc. III. Title.
RM666.P835E46 2007
615'.321—dc22

                                      2006022947

We dedicate this book to the volunteers who participated
in clinical trials for testing probiotics.
It is due to their encouragement that this book
was written and probiotic research has progressed.

CONTENTS

ABOUT THE AUTHORS

Gary W. Elmer, PhD, is Professor of Medicinal Chemistry at the University of Washington in Seattle. He is the co-author of *The Vitamin Book,* a consumer-oriented guide to vitamins.

Lynne McFarland, PhD, is a research health science specialist with the Puget Sound Veterans Administration, Health Services Research and Development, in Seattle, and was formerly Director of Scientific Affairs for an international pharmaceutical company that developed probiotics. Drs. Elmer and McFarland are globally recognized experts on probiotics and have been involved in the field for more than eighteen years. They have authored 37 original scientific articles on probiotics and co-edited *Biotherapeutic Agents and Infectious Diseases.* They have directed nine clinical trials evaluating a probiotic yeast and have lectured around the world on probiotics and their usefulness.

Marc McFarland, BS, is a writing and editing project specialist with the Prosthetic Research Study in Seattle. He was formerly Northwest News Editor/Bureau Manager for United Press International and special assistant to the Director of Scientific Affairs at Biocodex Inc., in Seattle.

Foreword

Probiotics are hot! You may ask yourself: What are probiotics? Most people have heard of antibiotics, but what are *probiotics*? The concept of probiotics dates to the early 1900s, when Nobel laureate Elie Metchnikoff theorized that the ingestion of beneficial microbes in dairy foods explained the relatively long life of Bulgarians, who regularly consume yogurt. Probiotics are living organisms that, when ingested, benefit the host. They have been used in many countries, especially in Europe, for many decades. Interest in the United States has been recently increasing with publication of information on controlled trials in diseases such as antibiotics-associated diarrhea and inflammatory bowel disease. With the increase in interest, a wide number of products is available, and over a thousand articles on probiotics have been published since 1990. But there are many questions. What are the products? What is their efficacy? What is the evidence of their usefulness? Who may benefit from their use?

Probiotics are especially appealing because they are a "natural" approach to treatment. Recently, very virulent strains of bacteria resistant to antibiotics have made the news. Use of nonantibiotic approaches to prevention and treatment is thus even more appealing.

This book addresses important clinical areas, including traveler's diarrhea, antibiotics-associated diarrhea, inflammatory bowel disease, irritable bowel disease, vaginitis, urinary tract infection, and allergies. Each chapter provides a summary of clinically relevant information, including traditional treatments. There is advice on when to use, when not to use, as well as the quality of probiotics.

This book is very welcome and timely. Written by well-established authorities in the field and an experienced journalist, it is an excellent review of probiotic use. The research data is extensively and thoroughly reviewed using evidence-based medicine rather than the

The Power of Probiotics
© 2007 by The Haworth Press, Inc. All rights reserved.
doi:10.1300/5597_a

"eminence-based," which has been the tradition. Although extremely detailed and precise, the writing is clear—a model of clarity, and the whimsical illustrations by Lynne McFarland add humor as well. The advice is practical and "no nonsense." In fact, the section on how to interpret a scientific study could benefit any reader interested in critical evaluation.

This book is a valuable resource for anyone interested in probiotics, and will be an excellent resource for health professionals as well.

Christina M. Surawicz, MD
Professor of Medicine,
University of Washington School of Medicine
and Chief of Gastroenterology,
Harborview Medical Center
Seattle, Washington

Preface

The impetus to write this book comes from the encouragement we have received from patients who volunteered to be part of our clinical trials for testing probiotics. Volunteers are very important to medical discoveries, as they often are the first people exposed to new medical treatments. Comments we usually received were, "These products are great!" "Why doesn't the general public know about them?" and "Why aren't more physicians and pharmacists recommending their use?"

Despite mounting and convincing evidence that probiotics are valuable in the prevention and treatment of some diseases, probiotics are relatively unknown to the public and underutilized by health professionals. Ask most people (even your physician) to describe probiotics, and it is likely you will get a blank stare. Part of the reason for this relative obscurity is the lack of useful information available to the consumer. Scientists and physicians have ready access to a vast literature base on probiotics. In the past decade alone, more than 1,000 research papers have been published with the term *probiotic* in the title. However, for the consumer, there is little by way of an easy to use, readable yet authoritative, and objective guide to probiotics.

This book fills that void. Each chapter discusses a disease or condition for which probiotics have been shown to be helpful. Each chapter starts with a question-and-answer section, and for some readers this may provide sufficient information to address their questions. The consumer wanting an in-depth discussion of a topic will find it in the text. Factual information is referenced so that the reader can pursue the subject even further, if desired. The relevant clinical studies and findings are summarized in easy-to-read tables, and each chapter contains a summary and recommendation section based on the in-depth discussion.

The Power of Probiotics
© 2007 by The Haworth Press, Inc. All rights reserved.
doi:10.1300/5597_b

xiii

A confusing variety of probiotics has appeared on store shelves, and Internet sites are full of health claims. How does a person separate the good information from the bad? How does one choose the right product? With probiotics, product selection is of paramount importance. Just as a specific drug is chosen for a specific medical condition, so should a specific probiotic be chosen for a specific ailment, and that selection should be based on evidence for effectiveness. This book has chapters to help select, from the myriad commercial products, the best probiotic to use for the treatment or prevention of specific medical conditions.

We believe this book is unique. Although there are a few other books about probiotics, they are targeted at the health professional and do not offer the scope of information that is found in this book. This book presents up-to-date information on probiotics in a way that is both quickly accessible and thoroughly in-depth. If you have a question, or many questions, about probiotics, we think you will find the answers in this book.

Acknowledgments

We would like to thank our fellow probiotics researchers for their tireless efforts to advance the understanding of these fascinating "living" drugs. We would also like to thank those who reviewed our chapters: Jackie Gardner, Lynn Imel, Lee Reid, Della Messer, Shan Goh, Melba McFarland, and Billy Joe McFarland. We extend our thanks to our friends and families for their support and patience during the writing of this book. And last, thanks to everyone who took part in the probiotic clinical trials over the years. Without your willing participation, beneficial discoveries cannot be made.

The Power of Probiotics
© 2007 by The Haworth Press, Inc. All rights reserved.
doi:10.1300/5597_c

Chapter 1

Introduction

This introductory chapter will discuss the basics of probiotics and what makes a good probiotic, and will provide some valuable tips on how to evaluate scientific studies for useful, practical information.

FREQUENTLY ASKED QUESTIONS

What are probiotics?

Probiotics are microorganisms (small, single-celled living organisms) that are ingested to benefit health and help fight diseases. Probiotics are either bacteria or yeasts.

Do bacteria and yeasts cause infections?

Indeed, disease-causing bacteria or yeasts (pathogens) can cause infections such as skin infections or pneumonia. Most other microorganisms are not harmful. Some microbes can even help maintain normal body functions and fight infections and diseases.

When are probiotics useful?

Probiotics can be helpful to prevent diarrhea while traveling or when taking antibiotics. Probiotics are useful for a wide variety of illnesses besides diarrhea. For chronic conditions, probiotics can be safely taken daily for years.

Are probiotics different from antibiotics?

Probiotics are living organisms taken for improving health. Antibiotics are substances that kill microorganisms. Antibiotics are "wonder drugs" for fighting infections, but they can have adverse effects (such as diarrhea, rashes, or allergic reactions). Some bacteria that cause infections have become resistant to treatment with common antibiotics. That leaves two choices: develop new antibiotics or come up with a different approach. Probiotics are that new approach.

Many different probiotic products are on the market today. Not all probiotic products or probiotic strains are the same. The types of bacteria or yeasts found in probiotic products may appear to be similar, but only some strains have been shown to be effective. This book will discuss the most effective strains so an informed choice can be made.

How do you know if a probiotic is really effective?

Marketing claims for probiotics are very diverse. Only those claims supported by well-conducted scientific studies should be trusted. Later in this chapter, we will discuss how to evaluate scientific studies.

Are probiotics regulated by the U.S. Food and Drug Administration (FDA) as are prescription drugs?

Yes and no. Yes, the FDA does keep track of probiotics as "dietary supplements," but no, the degree of oversight for effectiveness and safety is not as high as it is for prescription drugs. How this affects the consumer will be discussed in this chapter.

Where do you find probiotic products?

Since 1994, probiotics can be sold in the United States "over the counter" (without the need for a prescription) as "dietary supplements." Probiotic products can be found in pharmacies, as well as in some supermarkets and other stores (organic foods stores, supplement stores, and health food stores), or can be purchased on the Internet from many probiotics or health food Web sites. In many other countries, probiotics have been sold over the counter for many years.

Is "Acidophilus" a probiotic?

Yes, this is an example of one type of probiotic.

WHAT ARE PROBIOTICS?

Probiotic literally means "for life." Probiotics are small, single-celled, living organisms (microorganisms) that are ingested to benefit health and help fight diseases. Generally, probiotics are bacteria or yeasts. A wide array of different probiotics exists (see Figure 1.1), but most are bacteria of the *Lactobacillus, Bifidobacterium, Enterococcus,* or *Escherichia* genera or are yeasts of the genus *Saccharomyces.*

Do probiotics contain living bacteria?

Yes, and that is a good thing. There are billions of bacteria in the body helping in the digestion of food, producing vitamins, stimulating the immune system, and fighting infections. Most bacteria found in the human body are beneficial.

How are probiotics named? Just as larger organisms are. We humans are formally named *Homo sapiens,* for example. Microorganisms are referred to by their genus name, followed by a species name, which may be followed by a strain name. A genus group lumps together similar types of microbes (similar to a large family or clan). The species defines a narrower group (like members of a family with the same last name). Strains narrow it down to identical type organisms (much as people are identified by their first name). So, instead of identifying an individual by "Joe Smith of the Gardner clan," a microorganism would be named "*Gardner smith* strain Joe." An example is *Lactobacillus casei* strain Shirota. The genus and species names should be italicized.

The Gram stain is a useful way to characterize different types of bacteria. Bacteria either take up the purple stain (gram-positive) or

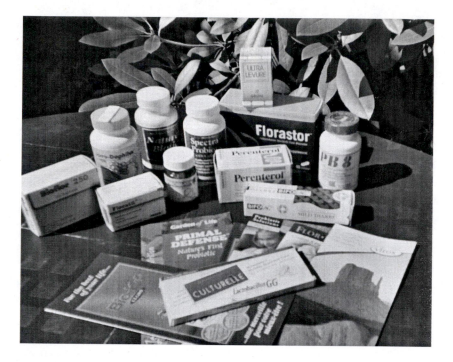

FIGURE 1.1. Examples of some current probiotic products are shown. *Source:* Photograph by Lynne V. McFarland.

not (gram-negative), and this is an easy first step in identifying bacteria. *Streptococcus pneumoniae* is an example of a gram-positive pathogen. *Escherichia coli* is gram-negative. The Gram stain appearances of these pathogens are shown in Figure 1.2.

- *The Gram stain was invented in 1884 by a Danish physician, Christian Gram*
- *Gram-positive microbes take up a crystal violet iodine stain, and the purple color cannot be washed out with alcohol*
- *Gram-negative microbes take up the stain, but alcohol wash removes the purple color*
- *The reason for the differential staining is due to fundamental differences between gram-positive and gram-negative cell walls*

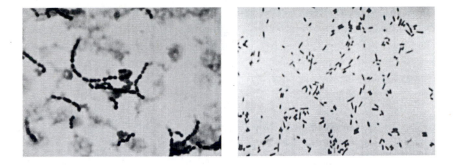

FIGURE 1.2. Gram stains of two different types of bacteria: On the left, *Strepto-coccus pneumoniae,* a gram-positive (purple stained) bacterium, and on the right, *Escherichia coli*, a gram-negative (red stained) bacterium. *Source:* Photograph by Lynne V. McFarland.

Probiotics are not antibiotics, chemicals, genetically altered foods, or artificial substances. They are living organisms that usually were first found in humans and then tested for their ability to fight or prevent disease. Probiotics are available in capsules, tablets, or a variety of food products. The probiotics sold in capsules usually are freeze-dried (lyophilized), which helps maintain their viability (number of living organisms) for extended periods of time. Some probiotics sold in capsules are heat-dried, liquid cultures of the probiotic, but the heating process used in the manufacturing of the product can kill the microbe and eliminate its probiotic benefit. Probiotics may be added to milk or other beverages. One example of a popular method for providing high probiotic activity is a yogurt containing living probiotic bacteria.

HISTORY OF PROBIOTICS

Probiotics are not something new invented in a laboratory. Microorganisms have been used for many centuries to preserve foods, although only in the previous century has the science of this process been understood. Early populations did not know that when they added a small amount of yogurt to the previous day's batch of milk and kept it in a warm place overnight they were seeding and propagating *Lactobacillus bulgaricus* and other lactic acid bacteria to coagulate milk protein. They knew only that the final product tasted good and lasted longer than raw milk. Other fermented foods have long been popular because of their taste and improved storage. For example, sauerkraut and kimchi result from bacterial action on cabbage (plus other vegetables for kimchi). Milk fermented by lactic acid-producing bacteria has long been thought to have more beneficial effects on health than milk itself. The heavy consumption of kefir by populations in the mountainous Caucasus region between the Black and Caspian seas has been associated with longevity, as has yogurt use in Bulgaria. Elie Metchnikoff (1845-1916), a Russian scientist, is credited with calling attention to the health benefits of yogurt. His hypothesis was that lactic acid bacteria in the yogurts counteract the harmful putrifying bacteria in the intestines. He associated the longevity of the Bulgarians and those from the Caucasus region with regular yogurt use and claimed to have improved his own ill health with sour milk fermented with lactic acid bacteria from Bulgaria. He credited his long life (71 years, long by the standards of his time) to ample amounts of yogurt in his diet, and his views were widely accepted at the time.[1]

In the early 1960s the term *probiotic* began to be applied to microbes used for medicinal purposes. A more recent and widely accepted definition is "defined, live microorganisms administered in adequate amounts, which confer a beneficial physiological effect on the host."[2] The use of probiotics has long remained popular in Europe and parts of Asia, but until recent years was uncommon in the United States. Today, probiotics are used worldwide, and the discovery of new, more effective probiotic microorganisms will serve to expand their medical applications. Nevertheless, few of the 1290 articles published on probiotics since 1990 are targeted for the general public. We hope this book will fill this gap.

MEDICAL CONDITIONS FOR PROBIOTICS

Not all diseases or conditions can be effectively treated with probiotics. Typically, diseases that respond best are those involving a disruption of normal microbial flora. The normal flora has a beneficial function, called "colonization resistance," that discourages pathogenic organisms from colonizing the body.[3] But this protective mechanism can be disrupted if the normal flora is disturbed by surgery, antibiotics, or other medications. Probiotic treatment can act as a substitute for these disturbed bacteria, or probiotics can produce substances that combat pathogenic bacteria and then work to restore the normal protective microflora.

What is normal microflora? Humans are normally host to billions of bacteria (see Figure 1.3). These bacteria help maintain many normal functions. A count of all the human cells would reveal that only

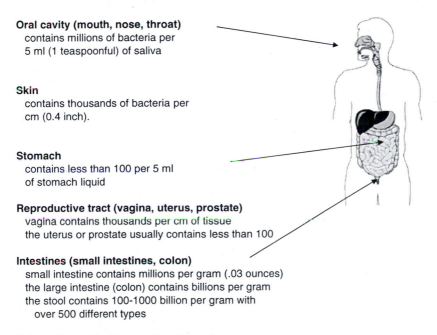

Oral cavity (mouth, nose, throat)
contains millions of bacteria per 5 ml (1 teaspoonful) of saliva

Skin
contains thousands of bacteria per cm (0.4 inch).

Stomach
contains less than 100 per 5 ml of stomach liquid

Reproductive tract (vagina, uterus, prostate)
vagina contains thousands per cm of tissue
the uterus or prostate usually contains less than 100

Intestines (small intestines, colon)
small intestine contains millions per gram (.03 ounces)
the large intestine (colon) contains billions per gram
the stool contains 100-1000 billion per gram with
   over 500 different types

Urinary Tract (bladder, urethra, kidney)

urethra contains less than 100 per cm of tissue
bladder and kidneys have none

FIGURE 1.3. Points where normal microflora is found in a healthy body are shown.

about 10 percent make up the body structure, while 90 percent are bacteria normally carried in or on the body. Most normal microflora is found in the gastrointestinal tract. There are millions of bacteria in the mouth, not very many in the stomach, and billions in the small and large intestines. All those bacteria are called "normal microflora." What is the function of normal microflora? Normal microflora has many important functions including helping to digest food, producing some vitamins, stimulating immune responses, and helping move food through the gastrointestinal tract. Normal flora also acts to protect against invasion by the ever-present, disease-causing bacteria we are exposed to. This defense mechanism is called "colonization resistance" because the layers of normal bacteria help form a barrier that resists colonization by pathogenic bacteria.

Several things can disrupt this protective colonization resistance. An antibiotic taken for an infection destroys the bacteria causing the illness, but it may also kill some of the beneficial microflora at the same time, leaving the person vulnerable to invasion by another pathogen once antibiotics are stopped. Most people can take antibiotics and recover from their illness before they are exposed to pathogenic bacteria that will take advantage of this opportunity. But if a person is hospitalized (which is an environment full of pathogenic bacteria) or is in a location that has poor quality water (for example, when traveling in some countries) or is already weakened due to chronic conditions, then such a person is at high risk of developing disease if the normal microflora is disrupted. It is in these types of situations and conditions that probiotics work best. Probiotics can help restore the normal protective flora and assist in other beneficial activities in the body.

Some diseases are caused by alterations to the normal microflora or to the body's response to normal microflora, but are not specifically caused by pathogenic overgrowth itself. These diseases may result from an imbalance in the immune response. Examples, which will be covered in later chapters, include inflammatory bowel disease, irritable bowel syndrome, Crohn's disease, and skin allergies. New research shows that probiotics can help restore the balance of normal microflora and help boost immune response. Some diverse conditions for which probiotics have been used are shown in Table 1.1.[4]

TABLE 1.1. Medical uses for probiotics.

Infectious diseases	Microbial imbalances	Other uses
Acute adult diarrhea	Constipation	Reduced stress effects
Antibiotic associated diarrhea	Kidney stones	Increased weight gain during development (veterinary use)
Helicobacter pylori dyspepsia and stomach ulcers	Chemotherapy induced diarrhea	Stabilization of normal flora
Pediatric diarrhea	Diabetes	Production of vitamins
Recurrent *Clostridium difficile* disease	Hypercholesteremia	Enhancing vaccine response
Nosocomial infections	Inflammatory bowel disease	Source of Vitamin B_{12}
Travelers diarrhea	Recolonization of the intestines after antibiotic treatment or surgery	Food allergies (lactose intolerance)
Urinary Tract Infections	Cancer	Stimulation of the immune system
Vaginitis	Irritable bowel disease	Atopic eczema
Vaginosis	Encephalopathy (liver disease)	Allergies
	Alcohol-induced liver disease	
	Enteral tube feeding-associated diarrhea	
	Pouchitis	
	Arthritis	

THE "IDEAL" PROBIOTIC

The ideal probiotic would possess numerous ways to fight pathogens, assist in restoring normal microflora, and have no adverse effects. Examples of desirable attributes for probiotics include:

- A stable and well-described microbe
- Lack of toxicity and pathogenicity
- Survives and perhaps multiplies in the location of desired action
- Persists in the host permanently
- Adheres to the target tissue
- Stimulates the immune system
- Synthesizes substances to combat infection
- Efficacy is proven in well-designed, placebo-controlled clinical trials

- Ease of large-scale commercial production and distribution
- Low cost for consumer purchase

Few probiotics currently meet all of these criteria. The road to achieving a probiotic that appeals to the public and has the support of the medical community is long and complex. For example, some researchers screened over 1,500 bacterial strains before finding a single strain that had probiotic potential.[5] After isolation, the probiotic strain must be carefully characterized so that it can be accurately described in the scientific literature. Then, lengthy studies need to be conducted in the laboratory (called "in vitro" studies) to test the new strain for stability and activity against pathogens or for other properties thought to be important for use in therapy. These in vitro studies are followed by studies in animal models of the disease. If these experiments show promise, then human volunteer studies (in vivo studies) are performed to define safety and the dose needed for a beneficial effect. These first clinical studies in humans are called Phase 1 clinical trials. Next, studies are conducted in patients, usually with a mild form of the disease, to get an idea of the extent of the benefits without unduly placing the patient at risk. These are called Phase 2 clinical trials. Finally, large-scale human studies (Phase 3 clinical studies) are undertaken in order to more carefully define the efficacy of the probiotic in patients with the disease indication.[6]

Useful properties of probiotics:

- *Survive in the human body*
- *Can kill pathogens*
- *Bind to human cells*
- *Stimulate the immune system*

Results from the Phase 3 clinical studies are of most importance in the decision of whether to try a probiotic to improve health. No matter how promising a probiotic may appear from its in vitro properties and from results in animal studies, if it does not work in people, it is of little interest. Unfortunately, there are many probiotic products on the market that have not been evaluated in well-designed and well-conducted clinical trials. Many may have some of the desirable properties listed here, but without the published results from human studies, the "proof" is not there to justify their purchase and use. In this book, detailed discussion and recommendations are focused on those probiotics that have been tested and found to be effective from testing in randomized, controlled, human clinical trials.

PROPERTIES OF CURRENT PROBIOTICS

A wide array of commercial probiotics is found on the market today. This can be confusing when trying to decide which one to purchase (see Figure 1.4). However, most products contain one or more similar probiotic microorganisms. The most common probiotic microbes found in commercial products are described in the following subsections.

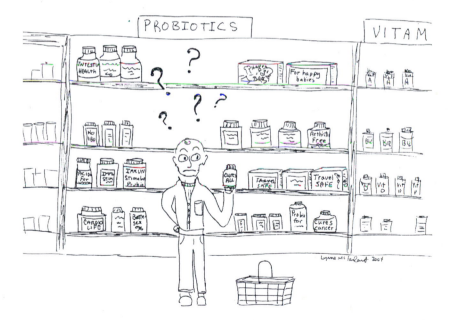

FIGURE 1.4. What exactly are probiotics? Confusion reigns at the store. *Source:* Illustration by Lynne V. McFarland.

Lactobacilli Species (General)

Lactobacilli have long been the most prominent probiotic microorganisms because of their association with popular fermented dairy products. Consumption of these products, such as yogurt, is commonly associated with good health. Lactobacilli are gram-positive rods and part of the large group of lactic-acid-producing bacteria. Lactobacilli are involved in pickling foods and making cheese and yogurt. Human strains of lactobacilli usually are part of the normal microflora in the mouth, lower small intestine, colon, and vagina. But they are not the dominant species in the intestinal tract. Fermentation of carbohydrates by lactobacilli produces lactic acid, so this type of bacteria survives well in acidic environments (such as in the stomach). This gives lactobacilli a competitive niche in environments rich in nutrients and may explain, in part, their probiotic action. They are rarely pathogenic.

Lactobacillus rhamnosus

Lactobacillus rhamnosus GG is the most studied lactobacilli probiotic. This strain of lactobacillus was isolated from the feces of a healthy human by two gastroenterologists, Drs. Sherwood Gorbach and Barry Goldin (hence, GG).[7] It has been variously designated *Lactobacillus casei* subspecies *rhamnosus* strain GG or *Lactobacillus rhamnosus* GG, but is commonly referred to as *Lactobacillus* GG. It is available from the American Type Culture Collection as *Lactobacillus* number ATCC 53103. *L. rhamnosus* GG is stable in bile and acid, and adheres to intestinal cells in vitro.[8] A substance produced from this strain kills a relatively broad spectrum of bacteria, but it is not known whether this antibacterial substance is produced when the probiotic is taken orally.[7]

How probiotics work:

Kill disease-causing bacteria
Destroy toxins
Boost antibodies
Form a barrier to disease-causing bacteria overgrowth
Interfere with disease process

L. rhamnosus GG survives passage through the stomach and intestinal tract. This was determined by analyzing stool samples from healthy adult volunteers receiving *L. rhamnosus* GG in fermented milk or whey for about a month. *L. rhamnosus* GG was recovered from stool while the probiotic was being taken and for about seven days after it was stopped.[8] Another study found *L. rhamnosus* GG in all intestinal biopsy and fecal samples 14 days after cessation of probiotic, but the lactobacilli disappeared 28 days after stopping ingestion.[9] There were more biopsy samples positive with *Lactobacillus* GG than positive fecal samples, indicating *L. rhamnosus* GG can adhere to, and perhaps divide on, the colonic mucosa.

Another useful property is modulation of specific enzymes by the probiotic. Feeding *L. rhamnosus* GG to healthy volunteers for four weeks decreased fecal β-glucuronidase-specific activity, whereas feeding *Streptococcus thermophilus* or *Lactobacillus bulgaricus* did not.[8] This enzyme may help prolong the time potential carcinogens are in the intestine. Lowering intestinal β-glucuronidase has the potential to decrease colon cancer. *L. rhamnosus* GG also was found to inhibit *Streptococcus sobrinus* (a bacterium involved in dental cavities)[10] and to colonize the mouth.[11]

Lactobacillus reuteri

Lactobacillus reuteri is another lactic-acid-producing bacterium with desirable probiotic properties. Strains of this microbe are widespread in nature and can be isolated from a variety of food products, animals, and the human gastrointestinal tract. In a laboratory setting (in vitro), *L. reuteri* produces several compounds that can destroy a wide variety of harmful bacteria. However, it is not clear whether these antimicrobial substances are produced in the human intestine in concentrations high enough to directly inhibit pathogens. *L. reuteri* appears to survive passage through the human digestive tract and persists for at least seven days after stopping ingestion. In a human study involving ingestion of this probiotic for 21 days, fecal samples from probiotic-treated volunteers contained significantly higher concentrations of *L. reuteri*, compared to placebo, from day 7 to 28, but not after 77 days.[12] Thus, some colonization was evident for at least seven days after cessation of dosing, but not at 30 days after stopping.

The probiotic activities of *L. reuteri* have been comprehensively reviewed.[13]

Lactobacillus acidophilus

Lactobacillus acidophilus is widespread in commercially available probiotic products. It is found in fermented dairy products, and is part of normal intestinal and vaginal microflora. However, properties of adherence and stability in the gastrointestinal tract are strain specific. Strains optimal for fermenting milk may not work well in the lower bowel or vaginal tract. Few direct comparisons of lactobacillus strains are published, so it is important to be clear about which strain is being investigated. *L. acidophilus* LCFM, a commonly used dairy strain, survives passage through the human gastrointestinal tract but does not colonize the intestines during two weeks consumption by healthy volunteers.[14] It was concluded that daily consumption is needed to maintain high intestinal levels of this probiotic strain. Several *L. acidophilus* strains have been shown to produce antimicrobial substances in vitro, but production in vivo (in the body) at levels high enough for a direct inhibition of pathogen growth has not been demonstrated. However, it seems that several strains of *L. acidophilus* have a number of desirable probiotic properties.

Lactobacillus casei

Similar to *Lactobacillus acidophilus,* the probiotic properties of *Lactobacillus casei* are strain specific. *L. casei* strain Shirota has received much commercial attention. It is effective against *E. coli* in mouse model for urinary tract infections,[15] against *Listeria monocytogenes* infections in rats,[16] reduces influenza virus titers in aged mice,[17] and reduces ulcer causing *Helicobacter pylori* in humans.[18] A placebo controlled trial showed an increase in fecal Bifidobacteria and a decrease in undesirable beta-glucuronidase and beta-glucosidase activities, but had no effect on the immune system in *L. casei* Shirota treated subjects.[19] This strain can favorably modify the composition and metabolic activities of human intestinal flora. It also survives passage through the human digestive tract.

Bifidobacteria Species

Bifidobacteria species are anaerobic lactic- and acetic-acid-producing bacteria. They are present in normal flora and are the major component in the intestinal flora of breast-fed infants. Upon weaning, levels of bifidobacteria decline. Bifidobacteria grow well in milk, and there has long been interest in bifidobacteria-containing probiotics in fermented dairy products. There is good evidence that several strains of bifidobacteria can survive passage through the gastrointestinal tract and may favorably affect intestinal functions. Recently, high fecal recovery (>10 percent of dose) was obtained in human volunteers receiving a *Bifidobacterium-breve*-fermented soy milk product.[20]

Enterococcus faecium

Another well-studied lactic-acid-producing probiotic is *Enterococcus faecium* SF68. Other strains of *Enterococcus faecium* are pathogenic and resistant to most antibiotics. Although strain SF68 is nontoxic, there has been concern that the probiotic might pick up and share antibiotic-resistant genes in the human gut. When given to humans, *Enterococcus faecium* SF68 was found in the feces at the end of oral dosing, but did not persist three weeks after the probiotic was stopped.[21]

Saccharomyces boulardii

Saccharomyces boulardii is a well-studied, commercially available yeast probiotic.[22] Unlike the lactobacilli, *S. boulardii* is not usually found in the gastrointestinal or vaginal tracts. However, it grows best at 37°C (normal human body temperature) and survives passage into the feces in both animals and humans.[23] The yeast does not strongly adhere to intestinal mucosa and is eliminated within one to three days if not readministered. It must be given daily to achieve effective levels. *S. boulardii,* being a yeast and not a bacterium, is not directly affected by antibacterial antibiotics, so it can be given simultaneously during antibiotic therapy. It would be adversely affected by antifungal therapy if is taken at the same time. One human study showed that fluconazole, a potent antifungal, did not reduce *S. boulardii* concentrations if the yeast and the antifungal dose were taken three hours apart.[24] *S. boulardii* produces a protease enzyme that degrades powerful toxins produced by the dangerous pathogen, *Clostridium difficile*.[25] This yeast also can stimulate the immune system[26] and increase the production of digestive enzymes in the intestinal mucosa.[27] All these properties make this yeast a useful probiotic.

HOW TO EVALUATE SCIENTIFIC STUDIES

Every day, it seems, there is news of a "breakthrough treatment" from yet another clinical study. The results often conflict what was said the day before. The results of different studies frequently do not agree with each other, even though they seem to be using the same drug or studying the same disease. All this can be quite confusing. The problem with depending on headlines or short articles for information is that they do not provide details on the quality of the study. It is important to be able to judge whether the claim for a medical product is based on solid science or shaky evidence.

Points to consider when evaluating scientific studies:

- *Study design*
- *Number enrolled*
- *Type of subject enrolled*
- *Follow-up*
- *How it was conducted*
- *Statistical significance*
- *Possible bias*
- *conclusion agrees with evidence*
- *consistent with other studies*
- *mechanism of action*

Consider these points when trying to evaluate a scientific study: the study design, the number of subjects enrolled, the types of subjects enrolled, how well the study was conducted, whether the result was statistically significant (i.e. the result was not due to chance), and if the conclusions agree with the evidence. When trying to decide if a probiotic or investigational treatment is effective, it also is important to compare the results of several studies, when possible. Are the results consistent between studies? How many studies have been conducted? Is there an explanation for how the treatment works (a mechanism of action)?

There are many types of study designs. Just because a study was conducted by a medical provider (physician, nurse, or pharmacist for example) it does not automatically mean one can depend on the results. The weakest studies to prove effectiveness are case reports (a description of one person's case), and case series (which summarize a small number of patients). These types of studies are valuable in that they can provide clues of promising treatments, but further research is needed to prove that the treatment is helpful for a significant number of people. Another type of study design is called an "uncontrolled" trial. This means there is no control (or comparison) group, that is, one that does not receive the study treatment. All the study subjects in an uncontrolled trial receive the treatment being tested. The problem with this type of design is one cannot be sure how many of the subjects would have improved without the investigational treatment. A more useful type of study uses an additional group called a "comparison" or "control" group. For diseases with common symptoms that have a tendency to get better by themselves given time (such as diarrhea), it is important to have a control group, which is not given the investigational treatment. The control group acts as a measure of what happens when the usual care is given. In a drug study, the control group would receive a placebo (an inert substance that is indistinguishable from the investigational treatment) or standard treatment (the usual care). This way, the rate of disease in the tested treatment group can be compared with the rate of disease in the control group. If there is no control group, the improvement of people who get better in the treatment group may be due to the tested medicine or may simply reflect what would have happened without any treatment.

Some types of studies are called "open studies." The type of treatment (investigational or the control) is not hidden or blinded from the patient or the people conducting the trial. This may lead to a biased assessment of the trial. Study volunteers who know which group they are assigned to tend to report illness more frequently if they know they are in the control group and, conversely, report less illness if they know they are in the investigational group. To minimize this type of bias, study treatments are often "blinded" or packaged in such a way that the type of assignment cannot be determined. The pills containing the investigational treatment and the control pills look the same.

The most valuable evidence comes from a study design called a "double-blind, randomized, controlled trial." In these studies, volunteers are enrolled, randomized (as in tossing a coin) into one of two treatment groups, and then followed-up for the study outcome. One group receives the active treatment that is being tested, and the other is the control group. If the study is double-blind, then neither the volunteers nor the scientists following the patients' progress know the true identity of the treatment given to each individual until after the study is completed (see Figure 1.5). This helps reduce any possible bias that might occur if the outcome is assessed by someone who

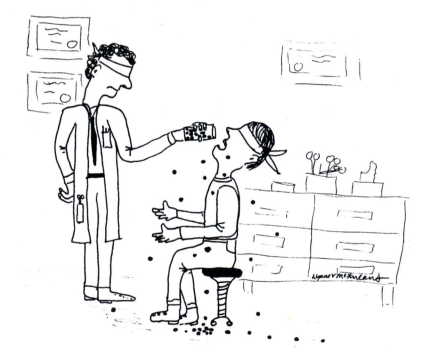

FIGURE 1.5. In a double-blind study, both the investigator and the study volunteer do not know which type of treatment the volunteer receives. *Source:* Illustration by Lynne V. McFarland.

knows which treatment was received. A double-blind, randomized, placebo-controlled study design gives the best chance that the result is due to the treatment being tested and not due to biases or errors in judgment or by chance alone.

It also is important to have sufficient numbers of subjects enrolled into a trial. A conclusion that a probiotic works is not on a very firm foundation if the study was conducted with only a few people. For example, one would have more confidence in a study conducted with 200 people as against 20, even though the findings from both studies were statistically significant (placebo versus treatment). The type of volunteers included in the trial is also important. Studies should explain the inclusion and exclusion criteria used. This gives an indication of how well the results of the trial can be generalized to other populations. For example, the findings from a study enrolling only young men may not be applicable to young women. How well a study was conducted also should be a consideration. If the investigators did not follow their protocol or if a large number of study subjects dropped out or were lost to follow-up, the results could be biased and the results may be erroneous.

Just because there was a difference in the cure rate between the treated group and the control group does not mean the the difference was meaningful. Only when the difference is "statistically significant" can it be concluded that the treatment had an effect. When results of trials are reported, it often is stated that the results were "statistically significant" and the authors will provide a p-value next to the result. What does this mysterious p-value mean? A difference between two groups can be due either to the treatment being tested or simply to random chance. Think of it this way: a coin being flipped in the air has a 50 percent chance of landing heads up, or a probability or p-value of 0.50. To be confident that the difference observed in the clinical trial is not merely due to chance variations in the study subjects, the p-value for significance should be set at an extremely low probability level. A widely accepted p-value for significance is 0.05 (or less). Therefore, "statistically significant" ($p = 0.05$) means the probability that the trial result was due to chance variations is less than 5 out of 100. Another point to consider is whether a conclusion drawn from the trial is supported by the evidence shown in the study. It is surprising how often authors may overstate the results of their clinical trials or ignore some findings if they were biased to find that the treatment would or would not work.

Once a study is completed, the results should be compared to other studies using the same investigational treatment. Are the results consistent from study to study? It is confusing when studies use the same treatment for the same disease and yet come to different conclusions. Differences in study design, the type of subjects enrolled, the severity of the disease, problems with bias, or failure to follow up can help explain these differing conclusions. To make a global judgment about whether a treatment works or not or to consider whether most of the studies agree with each other, look for a review article that analyzes the different studies and helps explain the different findings. Another factor is whether the study makes biological and clinical sense. Does the treatment have an explicable mechanism of the action of how it cures the disease? All these factors should be considered when evaluating the results and conclusions from clinical trials. In our recommendations for probiotic uses, we placed heavy reliance on those results coming from well-designed, randomized controlled studies conducted in humans.

REGULATIONS FOR PROBIOTICS

Regulations regarding probiotics vary from county to country. In the United States, probiotics are considered to be either foods or dietary supplements. Many foods use bacteria or fungi in the process of making the final product, but most bacteria or fungi are killed before they reach the last manufacturing step. Usually, this is done to stop the fermentation process and help extend the shelf life (length of time the food can last before it spoils). Often, the food or milk is pasteurized (heated) to reduce the numbers of bacteria and thus increase the shelf life. These types of foods (such as pasteurized cheese or milk) are not considered probiotics, even though some of the bacteria involved in the production of the food may be a strain that has been tested as a probiotic. As long as there are no living organisms present in the final product, no health or probiotic claims can be made. However, if a manufacturer chooses not to sterilize or pasteurize a product and the final product contains adequate amounts of living microorganisms and the strain used is a probiotic strain, then the food may be considered a "probiotic food." If the manufacturer makes no health claim on the product, then it is regulated under safe food regulations. An example of this is acidophilus milk, which is found in the dairy section of grocery stores and does not have any health claims on the product. Many European probiotics are manufactured and sold as probiotic foods (probiotics in yogurt, beverages, infant formulas, or cheeses). In the United States, most probiotics are not sold in foods; rather, they are sold as dietary supplements.

Dietary supplement health claim	*Prescription drug claim*
Enhances intestinal health	*Treats traveler's diarrhea*
Supports the immune system	*Treats inflammatory bowel disease*
Improves bone strength	*Treats osteopathy*
Maintains a healthy circulatory system	*Treats high blood pressure*

Dietary supplements are regulated differently from prescription drugs and over-the-counter medications, although all are ultimately regulated in the United States by the Food and Drug Administration (FDA). The FDA has strict policies for the development and labeling of prescription and over-the-counter medications. Years of research and clinical trials and, often, millions of dollars of development funds are necessary before a new investigational drug is approved by the FDA, and then the product can claim to only treat or cure the disease based on the studies submitted to the FDA. Over-the-counter medications also require considerable evidence from human clinical trials before FDA approval. In 1994, the Dietary Supplement Health and Education Act (DSHEA) was passed. Originally intended to allow some claims that vitamins could be useful for mild diseases (such as vitamin C and the common cold), this law allowed the door of opportunity to swing wide open for probiotics, herbals, and other natural products. Instead of having to go through the arduous path of FDA approval, substances regulated as dietary supplements could be sold in the United States with very limited health claims on the label. Dietary supplements do not need to use multimillion dollar clinical trials to prove to the FDA that they work against specific diseases.

However, the manufacturer is limited in what can be said on the product label. Dietary supplements are not allowed to claim that they "treat" or "prevent" a specific disease, such as "treats cancer" or "prevents diarrhea." They can make only what are referred to as "structure or function health claims."[28] These include milder statements of effectiveness, such as "enhancing normal functioning," "leads to well-being," or "helps maintain health." To make structure/function claims on a product label, manufacturers must have some substantiation that the statements are truthful and not misleading. In 1998, DSHEA was revised such that manufacturers could not use signs or symptoms of a disease in a health claim (such as "lowers cholesterol" or "lowers blood glucose") and the name of the dietary supplement cannot imply a treatment or cure (such as "Cardiotabs"). The product also must bear the following disclaimer: "This statement has not been evaluated by the Food and Drug Administration. This drug is not intended to diagnose, treat, cure, or prevent any disease." Manufacturers of dietary supplements do not have to submit substantiation of their claim before they market their product, but they do have to notify the FDA of their health claim within 30 days of introducing their product to market. The FDA does not routinely ask for claim substantiation.

Dietary supplements also must have ingredient labeling on the product (name and quantity of each dietary ingredient), and the label must identify the product as a dietary supplement. Labels also must provide nutrition information, which lists ingredients present in significant amounts. Although not specifically required by law, most probiotics should state the dose and potency (the number of living microorganisms contained per capsule or per weight of product). Microbiologists deal in large numbers: because millions of bacteria can be present on the point of a pin, common doses of probiotics taken on a daily basis usually consist of several billion living microbial cells. Often the potency of a probiotic product will be expressed in billions per capsule or written as "10^9 per capsule." Rarely a "log value" of "log 9 per capsule" may be stated on the label. Just remember that 1 billion is the same as 10^9 or log 9. Normally, a dose of at least 1 billion living microorganisms per day is needed to achieve a therapeutic effect. A label may also state "10^9 cfu per capsule." The abbreviation "cfu" stands for "colony-forming units," or the number of colonies that grow when it is cultured in a microbiology laboratory. The cfu indicates how many living organisms are contained in the probiotic (one organism = 1 cfu).

Dietary supplements must be safe and unadulterated. A product is considered unsafe if one of its ingredients presents a significant or unreasonable risk of illness or injury. It is considered adulterated if a major ingredient is not listed on the product label. Currently, there are no good manufacturing practices (GMPs) for dietary supplements. GMPs are required for prescription drugs and over-the-counter medications, and involve detailed manufacturing protocols and FDA inspections of the manufacturing plants. Overall, dietary supplements are not as closely regulated as prescription and over-the-counter drugs, but so far, the safety of probiotics has been excellent.

With the regulations in mind, it is prudent to compare the health claims listed on the label of a probiotic with what is allowed for your country. As regulations vary between countries, this may be difficult. This will be covered in a later chapter describing various probiotic products. However, one simple rule can be used as a guide. If the health claims seem exaggerated or far-fetched, or cover a wide variety of diseases, they probably are not true. No probiotic has been scientifically proven to cure cancer or restore hair loss (yet). So, if a probiotic states it can, one can be sure that the manufacturer or marketer is not being truthful.

Responsible manufacturers of probiotics do their best to abide by the regulations and claim only what is reasonable based on available evidence and what is allowed by law. In the purchase of probiotics on the Internet, be aware that the health claims may not reflect the country where you live; rather, the health claims reflect the regulations of the country from which the probiotic is being sold.

THE FUTURE OF PROBIOTICS

As the effectiveness of antibiotics becomes less certain due to antibiotic resistance, the role for probiotics may become much stronger. Probiotics offer a unique ability to work with the natural body systems to improve health and, at the same time, to fight pathogenic organisms in multiple ways. However, as information in this book will show, not all strains of probiotics are effective for all diseases or conditions. For example, *Lactobacillus rhamnosus* is a probiotic that is effective for pediatric diarrhea and allergies, but does not appear to be effective for inflammatory bowel disease. In the future, specific probiotics may be developed for specific disease conditions. For example, genetic engineering can be used to enhance the expression of genes that code for proteins that neutralize specific toxins. Other genes that code for molecules that stimulate the immune system could be targeted. Genetic engineering could be used to enhance the production of beneficial enzymes that help combat diseases. Genetic tools could also be used to engineer probiotic strains that could serve as vaccines.

Another future direction for probiotics may be better selection of strains that have desirable properties. Strains of probiotics that are better colonizers of the human body, can adhere to cellular surfaces, survive during transit through the body, have useful metabolic products, and have pathogen-destroying enzymes will be important properties on which to focus for selection. Specific strain selection to target specific diseases will help bring probiotics into mainstream medicine in the future.

Chapter 2

Traveler's Diarrhea

Bacterial and viral diarrheas, including traveler's diarrhea, are leading causes of disease and death throughout the world. The consequences of traveler's diarrhea include dehydration, disruption of a trip (either vacation or business trips), and economic losses for tourists and insurance companies and for tourist-related industries (hotels, airlines, attractions, cruise lines, etc.) due to cancelled or shortened trips. Use of probiotics for traveler's diarrhea is safe and effective.

FREQUENTLY ASKED QUESTIONS

Who gets traveler's diarrhea?

Traveler's diarrhea is the most common illness affecting travelers. Each year, up to half of all international travelers (an estimated 10 to 12 million people worldwide) develop traveler's diarrhea. One out of four tourists who develop traveler's diarrhea has to change travel plans in some way.

What are the common symptoms of traveler's diarrhea?

Most cases begin abruptly with diarrhea, usually between four and five loose bowel movements per day. Other common symptoms are abdominal cramping, nausea, vomiting, malaise, and bloating.

The Power of Probiotics
© 2007 by The Haworth Press, Inc. All rights reserved.
doi:10.1300/5597_02

Where are the high-risk areas for traveler's diarrhea?

Areas of high risk include Africa, the Middle East, Latin America, and Asia.

Is not "Montezuma's revenge" just an annoyance and not very serious?

Usually traveler's diarrhea lasts just for a few days. However, diarrhea can be prolonged in some cases, and can be dangerous for the frail and for young children. Traveler's diarrhea can disrupt your trip, result in more severe illness, or, at the very least, alter your view during your vacation (see Figure 2.1).

Can it not be avoided by drinking bottled water?

Travelers often become ill due to unsuspected sources. Consumption of ice in beverages, food from street vendors, and cold salads can result in traveler's diarrhea.

What about cruise ships?

When an outbreak of viral traveler's diarrhea occurs on a cruise ship, large numbers of travelers can be simultaneously affected.

Why not rely on Pepto-Bismol?

The effective dose of Pepto-Bismol is six to eight tablets per day. For a two-week trip this constitutes 112 tablets. Pepto-Bismol should be avoided by those allergic to salicylates.

Why not take antibiotics to prevent traveler's diarrhea?

Antibiotics should be used only for treatment and not for prevention of traveler's diarrhea.

Are probiotics safe to take for the duration of the trip?

Unlike most medications and antibiotics used for traveler's diarrhea, prolonged use of probiotics is safe.

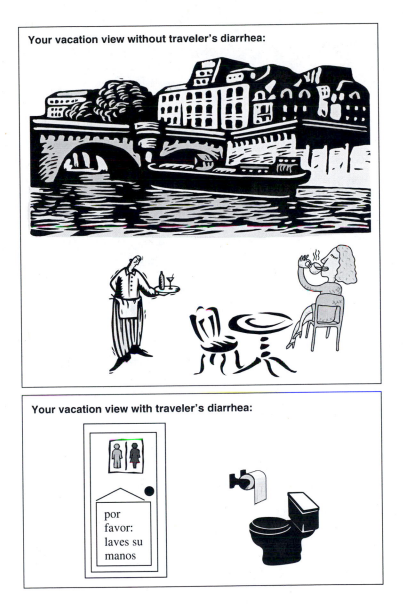

FIGURE 2.1. View of your vacation with and without traveler's diarrhea.

Are probiotics effective in preventing traveler's diarrhea?

Several probiotics have been shown by scientific studies to be safe and effective for the prevention of traveler's diarrhea.

RISKS FOR TRAVELER'S DIARRHEA

Diarrhea is the most common health problem among travelers (with the possible exception of sunburn). Every year 12 million cases of traveler's diarrhea are reported.[1] Depending on the destination, rates for traveler's diarrhea vary from areas of high incidence (over 50 percent) to those of low incidence (5 to 10 percent).[2] The destinations can be broken down into three risk groups as shown in Table 2.1. High-risk destinations include northern Africa, Latin America, the Middle East, and Southeast Asia.[3,4] In one study of 784 American tourists traveling to developing countries, nearly half reported they developed diarrhea during their trip.[5] Intermediate-risk destinations include most of southern Europe, Israel, Japan, South Africa, and most of the Caribbean. In one study, of the 12,499 tourists leaving Brazil, 1675 (13.4 percent) reported to have developed traveler's diarrhea during their stay.[3] Low-risk destinations include North America, northern Europe, Australia, New Zealand, and the United Kingdom. However, it is worth noting that traveler's diarrhea can strike even "presumed safe" destinations.

One out of four tourists may develop traveler's diarrhea

TABLE 2.1. Geographic areas by risk of traveler's diarrhea.

High-risk destinations (30-50%)	Intermediate-risk destinations (11-29%)	Low-risk destinations (5-10%)
Northern Africa	Southern Europe	North America
Latin America	Brazil	Northern Europe
Middle East	Israel	United Kingdom
Southeast Asia	Japan	Australia
	South Africa	New Zealand
	Caribbean	

Source of Traveler's Diarrhea

Traveler's diarrhea is acquired by ingestion of contaminated food, water, or other liquids. Both cooked and uncooked food may be risky if improperly handled or stored. High-risk foods include raw or undercooked meats and seafood, and unpeeled raw fruits and vegetables. Tap water, ice, unpasteurized milk, and other diary products are high risk. Tourists often forget that the ice in a drink (thought to be safe like bottled water) or the tap water used to brush their teeth may be a source for traveler's diarrhea. The riskiest sources of contaminated food are street vendors, farmers markets, and small restaurants.[6]

Foods are not usually suspected of harboring disease-causing bacteria, which are frequently the cause of a traveler's illness. Tests of Mexican-style condiments (green and red sauces, guacamole, and *pico de gallo*) at two restaurants found that 66 percent of the sauces at a Guadalajara, Mexico, restaurant and 40 percent of the sauces at a Houston, Texas, restaurant were contaminated with bacteria that can cause traveler's diarrhea.[7] Table 2.2 presents the types of foods and beverages that should be used with caution.

TABLE 2.2. Dietary advice regarding traveler's diarrhea.

High risk	Intermediate risk	Low risk
Foods		
Buffets or market foods kept at room temperature	Foods kept warm	Buffets or market foods kept hot
Rare hamburger or meat	Medium-cooked	Well-done meat
Unpeeled fruits or vegetables	Hamburger or meat	Peeled or cooked vegetables
Unpasteurized milk or butter	Cold salads	Peeled fruits
Fresh soft cheeses	Dry foods	Processed or packaged salads or foods
Shellfish (scallops, mussels, oysters, and clams)		Well-cooked eggs
Raw or runny eggs		
Condiment sauces left on tables		
Drinks		
Ice from unknown source	Ice made from potable water source	Boiled or iodized water
Tap water	Bottled fruit juices	Bottled water or beverages
Fruit juices from vendors or markets		

Symptoms and Complications

The incubation period (time from exposure to the contaminated food or liquid to the beginning of symptoms) usually is two to three days. The major symptom is diarrhea (four to six loose, watery, or bloody bowel movements per day).[8] The duration of traveler's diarrhea usually is two to six days, if untreated.[3] Other common symptoms are abdominal cramps and nausea. Vomiting and fever are less common.[6] If a traveler experiences vomiting two to four hours after a meal and does not develop diarrhea, the illness is probably food poisoning due to *Staphylococcus aureus,* not traveler's diarrhea.

In up to 15 percent of cases, diarrhea may be prolonged (one week to one month or, rarely, up to one year) and may be associated with repeated bouts of abdominal cramping, malaise, nausea, fever, or muscle pain. Travelers also may experience more than one episode of traveler's diarrhea during a single trip. Traveler's diarrhea may be especially hazardous for children and in people who are frail or immunocompromised because of severe dehydration.[9]

Consequences of Traveler's Diarrhea

Traveler's diarrhea often is thought of as just a day or two of inconvenience. However, traveler's diarrhea causes changes in travel plans (35 percent of 784 surveyed tourists), economic losses to the traveling public (cancelled trips, delays, and changed tickets), and economic losses to the host country and its tourist-related industries.[5] In addition, when the affected tourist is a child or someone frail or immunocompromised, the resulting dehydration can be life threatening.

Vulnerable Populations

Traveler's diarrhea usually is experienced by individual travelers, but outbreaks of traveler's diarrhea involving large groups of people also occur. Most at risk are groups visiting developing countries, passengers on cruise ships, Peace Corps or other voluntary health teams, and military personnel on overseas missions.[6,10-14] In North America, 4.5 million tourists travel by cruise ships each year.[12] The frequency of traveler's diarrhea outbreaks has increased from 1 in every 1,000 cruises during 1996 to 4 to 6 outbreaks in every 1,000 cruises in

2004.[14] The number of reported outbreaks also has increased dramatically, from 3 per year in the 1990s to 24 per year in 2002 and 30 in 2003.[6] In the late 1990s, outbreaks on cruise ships usually were foodborne (seafood), but outbreaks of Norwalk virus cause most of the outbreaks on cruise ships today.[6,10,14] Waterborne outbreaks caused by bacterial pathogens have been reported when beverages were made with ice from suspect sources, such as water that is not bottled or pumped in from local sources and not treated on the ship.[13]

Outbreaks of traveler's diarrhea can occur if groups are traveling together and there is a common source, such as contaminated water. Outbreaks also can occur if the organism spreads by person-to-person contact or through the air. Cruise ship outbreaks demonstrate how easily these viruses can be transmitted in a closed environment, affecting large numbers of tourists. In 2000, 21 outbreaks of traveler's diarrhea on cruise ships were investigated, with an average of 300 people ill per cruise.[6,10] This is an important health concern. If as few as 3 percent of passengers on a cruise ship develop traveler's diarrhea, the federal government is required to investigate. Information about outbreaks and safety profiles of various cruise ships can be accessed on the Centers for Disease Control and Prevention Web site (www.cdc.gov/travel).

Other groups can be at high risk for traveler's diarrhea. Peace Corps volunteers may be particularly susceptible. Among 4,607 Peace Corps volunteers serving in 43 different countries, 9 in 1,000 per year developed traveler's diarrhea, with the highest rates (33 percent) observed in Haiti, Central and West Africa, and Nepal.[15] Traveler's diarrhea is the most common prevalent medical condition (29 percent) in combat military troops on short-term missions.[11]

Risk Factors for Traveler's Diarrhea

Traveler's diarrhea is more common in young adults than older people. The reason for this is unclear, but may reflect a lack of acquired immunity, more adventurous travel styles, and different eating habits and behaviors that may involve increased risk from contaminated foods and liquids. A survey of 12,499 tourists leaving Brazil found an increased risk of developing traveler's diarrhea in the following:

- Age less than 36 years
- Male gender
- Length of trip
- Being a tourist, not a business traveler[3]

Another survey of 869 tourists traveling to various developing countries found these factors carried a high risk of traveler's diarrhea:

- Travel to northern Africa (59 percent became ill)
- Travel to India (56 percent became ill)
- Duration of travel (56 percent traveling more than 30 days became ill)
- Children of ten years of age or younger[5]

Etiologies (Causes) of Traveler's Diarrhea

Most (80 to 85 percent) cases of traveler's diarrhea are due to bacterial pathogens (enterotoxigenic *Escherichia coli*, enteroaggregative *E. coli*, *Campylobacter jejuni*, *Shigella* species, *Salmonella* species, *Vibrio parahemolyticus*, *Plesiomonas shigelloides*, *Aeromonas hydrophila*, *Yersinia enterocolitica*, and *Vibrio cholerae*). The most common cause of bacterial traveler's diarrhea is one of the seven types of diarrheagenic *E. coli*.[16,17] One symptom of traveler's diarrhea caused by *E. coli* usually is watery bowel movements associated with cramps. Fever typically is low grade or absent. When the cause of traveler's diarrhea was determined in 636 travelers from the United States, Canada, or Europe, 26 percent were because of one type of *E. coli*.[17]

Bacteria other than *E. coli* can cause traveler's diarrhea. *Salmonella* gastroenteritis occurs around the world and usually is associated with contaminated foods. *Salmonella* can cause dysentery (diarrhea with blood and mucus) with small-volume stools. *Vibrio parahemolyticus* is associated with the ingestion of raw or poorly cooked seafood (clams, mussels, oysters, and certain types of fish). Outbreaks of traveler's diarrhea caused by these bacteria have been reported on cruise ships in the Caribbean and Asia.[6] *Campylobacter jejuni* or *Campylobacter coli* are leading causes of traveler's diarrhea, especially in Thailand. This bacterium caused over half the diarrhea found in military troops sent to Thailand. Antibiotic resistance to ciprofloxacin was found in 96 percent of the bacteria tested.[18] Infections due to *Campylobacter* may be more severe than the usual case of traveler's diarrhea, with a higher rate of fever (65 percent), muscle weakness (53 percent), joint pain (47 percent), and duration of diarrhea (an average of 3.2 days).[18]

Other less frequent causes of traveler's diarrhea are viruses (Norwalk or rotavirus) and parasites (*Entamoeba histolytica, Giardia lamblia, Cyclospora,* and *Cryptosporidium*). Sometimes the cause cannot be determined. Not all types of bacteria, viruses, or parasites can be identified by current laboratory tests. In fact, some traveler's diarrhea may not result from an infectious organism at all, but simply is due to stress, jet lag, altitude, fatigue, or changes in diet.

PREVENTION OF TRAVELER'S DIARRHEA

The best strategy to prevent traveler's diarrhea is education and avoiding contaminated foods and liquids. As easy as this sounds, most tourists do not follow these guidelines.[3] Their focus usually is on their vacation and not food safety. Tourists often engage in riskier behaviors at exotic destinations than at home. Interestingly, business travelers have a lower rate of traveler's diarrhea than tourists. They may be more cautious and are more likely to get meals at their hotel and not from a street vendor.[19] The most effective strategy is to prevent exposure to the bacteria or viruses that can cause illness. "Boil it, cook it, peel it, or forget it" sums up the best strategy to prevent traveler's diarrhea (see Figure 2.2).

Medications

The most common medication recommended for traveler's diarrhea is bismuth subsalicylate (BSS). BSS (the active ingredient in Pepto-Bismol) is best when taken with food four times daily.[20] Prolonged use over three weeks is not recommended.[6] BSS should not be used when taking oral anticoagulants (blood thinners), as the typical dose of BSS acts as an equivalent of three to four aspirin. BSS should not be used when taking some types of antibiotics such as tetracyclines or fluoroquinolones. BSS should be avoided by those who are allergic to aspirin, have kidney problems or gout, children with chicken pox or flu (due to the potential risk of Reye's syndrome), and chil-

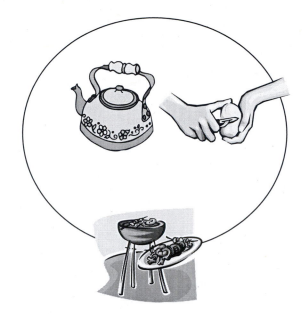

FIGURE 2.2. Behaviors to prevent traveler's diarrhea: Boil it, peel it, cook it, or forget it.

dren under the age of three years. Adverse effects of BSS include black stools, black tongue (the mouth should be rinsed after taking BSS), occasional nausea and constipation, and, rarely, tinnitus, also known as "ringing in the ears." BSS frequently does not work to prevent traveler's diarrhea simply because people on vacation do not follow label directions to take a full dose of six to eight tablets per day.

Antibiotics

Prophylactic antibiotic use is not recommended. Although some antibiotics are effective in reducing almost half the cases of traveler's diarrhea, other concerns outweigh their usefulness.[6] Trimethoprim/sulfamethoxazole (TMP/SMX), doxycycline, and fluoroquinolones (including ciprofloxacin) are the most commonly used antibiotics. Ciprofloxacin given frequently to travelers is 90 percent effective, but should not be used by women who are pregnant or be given to children. The problem with relying on antibiotics to prevent traveler's diarrhea is that they are effective for only a narrow range of bacteria. If a person develops traveler's diarrhea, the cause may be due to a virus or parasite, which the antibiotic may not target, or a strain of bacteria that is resistant to the antibiotic.

Another reason not to use antibiotics as a preventive therapy is that the cause of traveler's diarrhea usually is not known, making targeted antibiotic selection difficult. Furthermore, overuse leads to antibiotic resistance, which is increasing worldwide. Also, antibiotics are not without adverse effects. Prolonged use of antibiotics can create an opportunity for harmful resistant bacteria to multiply and cause other types of infections, which are called "overgrowth syndromes" (for example, *Candida* vaginitis, *Clostridium difficile* colitis) that may be more serious than traveler's diarrhea itself.[21,22] Use of antibiotics causes complacency, or a false sense of security, that may lead the traveler to engage in high-risk behaviors. The CDC does not recommend prophylactic antibiotics for traveler's diarrhea.[6]

Probiotics

With concerns over the costs of antibiotic treatments, emerging new cases of diseases, and the increasing frequency of antibiotic resistance, newer strategies for the prevention of traveler's diarrhea are needed. One of the most promising is the use of probiotics for the prevention of various types of diarrhea.[23,24] Use of probiotic microorganisms lowers dependence on antibiotics, is relatively inexpensive, and is well tolerated, even in prolonged use.

One of the reasons tourists become susceptible to illness is that travel can disrupt the body's normal defense mechanisms against infections. Stress, jet lag, unfamiliar foods and water, and disrupted body rhythms can disturb the normally protective bacteria in the intestines. These protective bacteria usually fight off disease-causing bacteria and viruses by "colonization resistance" (see Figure 2.3). Colonization resistance is a barrier effect that prevents attachment and colonization by harmful microorganisms.[23] It relies on the cooperation of different types of normal bacteria in the intestinal tract. The advantage of this type of defense is that it does not rely on one narrow range of targets (the way antibiotics do), but has multiple methods to

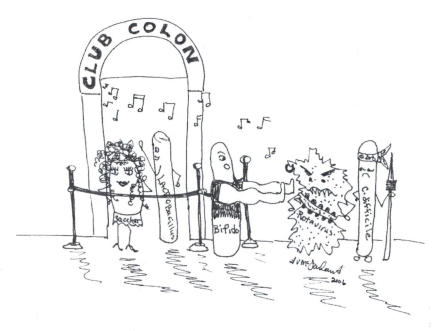

FIGURE 2.3. Colonization resistance is a natural defense mechanism by the normal microflora. Members of the intestinal flora (for example, *Bifidobacterium*) act as bouncers and do not let pathogens (for example, rotavirus or *Clostridium difficile*) colonize the intestines. When the normal flora is disrupted, probiotics, such as *Saccharomyces boulardii* or *Lactobacillus acidophilus*, can help keep pathogens at bay until the normal flora has recovered. *Source:* Illustration by Lynne V. McFarland.

deter harmful bacteria. These mechanisms are covered in other chapters of this book, but, briefly, they include:

- Production of antimicrobial substances that kill the harmful bacteria
- Production of enzymes that destroy or deactivate disease-producing toxins
- Stimulation of the immune system to produce more protective antibodies
- Competitive inhibition, which blocks pathogen attachment sites in the colon

Probiotics act as a "buffer" in inhibiting the growth of harmful bacteria while allowing the normal protective intestinal microflora to recover from the effects of travel and restore colonization resistance. Probiotics protect during these susceptible times. Traveler's diarrhea is the most common reason Europeans take probiotics. Although several types of probiotics have been tested for prevention of traveler's diarrhea (see Table 2.3), only three probiotics have been subject to rigorous scientific study.

TABLE 2.3. Probiotics used for the prevention of traveler's diarrhea.

Probiotic	Number in study	Population and destination	Frequency of traveler's diarrhea		
			Probiotic	Placebo	Reference
Saccharomyces boulardii	1,016	Austrian tourists to various locations	34%* (250 mg/day) 29%* (1 g/day)	39%	Note 25
Saccharomyces boulardii	1,231	Austrian tourists to hot climates	34%* (250 mg/day) 32%* (500 mg/day)	43%	Note 26
Lactobacillus acidophius	319	Austrian tourists to hot climates	53% NS	47%	Note 26
Lactobacillus acidophilus	282	British soldiers to Belize	26% NS	24%	Note 27
Lactobacillus rhamnosus GG	756	Finnish tourists to Turkey	41% NS	46.5%	Note 28
Lactobacillus rhamnosus GG	245	American tourists to various locations	3.9%*	7.4%	Note 29
Lactobacillus. fermentum	282	British soldiers to Belize	24% NS	24%	Note 27
Mixtures					
Lactinex (L. Acidophilus and L. bulgaricus)	50	American tourists to Mexico	35% NS	29%	Note 30
L. Acidophilus and Bifidobacterium bifidum and Streptococcus thermophilus	94	Danish tourists to Egypt	43%*	71%	Note 31

*$p < 0.05$; probiotic was significantly more effective than placebo.

NS = not significant.

Saccharomyces boulardii

Saccharomyces boulardii is a lyophilized (freeze-dried) yeast and packaged in capsules that are taken by mouth (Ultra-Levure, Parenterol, Florastor; Laboratoires Biocodex, Montrouge, France). It is widely available in Europe, South America, Africa, Sweden, and Mexico. In the United States, it is available as a dietary supplement (Florastor). This yeast is nonpathogenic and has been used to treat diarrhea while maintaining an excellent reputation for safety. *S. boulardii* achieves high concentrations in the intestine within three to four days, does not permanently colonize the intestine or translocate (leave the intestine for other body tissues), and is quickly cleared from the colon (within four to six days) after the yeast has been discontinued.[32]

In a large study, prevention of traveler's diarrhea was investigated among 1,016 Austrian tourists traveling to northern Africa, the Middle East, and Far East.[25] Tourists were given either a low dose of *Saccharomyces boulardii* (250 mg/day), a high dose of *Saccharomyces boulardii* (1 g/day), or a placebo, then diarrheal symptoms were recorded. *S. boulardii* significantly reduced traveler's diarrhea in a dose-dependent manner. Patients treated with placebo had a higher frequency (39 percent) of traveler's diarrhea compared to both the low dose (34 percent) and the high dose of *S. boulardii* (29 percent) groups. No significant side effects were reported. Another large study was conducted in 1,231 Austrian tourists traveling to hot climates. Traveler's diarrhea developed in 43 percent given placebo, but in significantly fewer tourists given either 250 mg/day (34 percent) or 500 mg/d (32 percent) of *Saccharomyces boulardii.*[26] More double-blinded, placebo-controlled trials are necessary to define the extent of protective action of *S. boulardii,* but the results published to date show promise.

Lactobacilli Probiotics

Several *Lactobacillus* species have been studied for prevention of traveler's diarrhea (Table 2.3), including *Lactobacillus rhamnosus* strain GG, *Lactobacillus acidophilus,* and *L. fermentum.*[26-29,33] *Lactobacillus rhamnosus* GG, originally isolated in humans, is resistant to bile and acid, binds to intestinal cells, produces several microbe-fighting substances, and has been studied in blinded clinical trials.[34] *Lactobacillus rhamnosus* GG usually is taken as powder contained within a capsule or as a fermented milk product (Gefilus, Valio Dairies, Helsinki, Finland). *Lactobacillus* GG is widely available. In the United States, it is sold as a dietary supplement (Culturelle).

Five blinded, controlled trials have been conducted with a lactobacillus-containing probiotic. In one study of 319 tourists, *Lactobacillus acidophilus* (2×10^9 organisms/day) or placebo was given to the tourists and they were asked to report if they developed traveler's diarrhea during their trip.[26] Traveler's diarrhea occurred as frequently in the tourists treated with *L. acidophilus* (53 percent) as those given placebo (47 percent).

Another study was conducted in 1990 with 820 Finnish travelers going to one of two cities in Turkey.[28] They were given either *L. rhamnosus* GG (2×10^9 organisms/day) or placebo in daily packets, and during the plane ride home, 756 completed a questionnaire about any illnesses during their trip. Overall, 41.0 percent given *L. rhamnosus* GG and a similar number given placebo developed traveler's diarrhea (46.5 percent, $p = 0.06$). Interestingly, the effect of the probiotic was more pronounced in one city than the other. Among tourists going to Alanya, Turkey, for one week, 17 (23.0 percent) given *L. rhamnosus* GG developed traveler's diarrhea, while significantly more 30 (39.5 percent) given placebo developed diarrhea ($p = 0.04$). (Refer to Chapter 1 for an explanation of statistical significance and *p*-values.) In the tourists going to Marmaris, Turkey, 68 (38.9 percent) given *L. rhamnosus* GG and 74 (42.3 percent) given placebo developed traveler's diarrhea, which were not significantly different. No side effects related to the probiotic were reported. This study did not propose a reason why *L. rhamnosus* GG seemed to work in one city and not the other, but this may have been due to different pathogens in the areas or because the placebo group going to Marmaris was slightly older.

Another study was conducted with 245 adult patients seen at a travel and immunization center who were traveling from the United States to developing countries for one to three weeks.[29] Tourists were randomly assigned to either *L. rhamnosus* GG (2×10^9 organisms/ day) or placebo to take during their stay. The risk of developing traveler's diarrhea was significantly lower in the group taking *L. rham-*

nosus GG (3.9 percent) compared to the group taking placebo (7.4 percent, $p = 0.05$). No serious side effects were observed in the treatment group.

Probiotic Mixtures

Based on the concept that the healthy colon functions effectively due to the multiple types of normal microflora residing within, another tactic has been tried using mixtures of different probiotic strains, instead of relying upon a single type of bacteria or yeast. A group of 50 travelers going to Mexico was randomized to either Lactinex (a mixture of *Lactobacillus acidophilus* and *Lactobacillus bulgaris*) or placebo for one week.[30] There was no significant difference in the frequency of traveler's diarrhea in the group given the probiotic mixture (35 percent) and those given placebo (29 percent).

However, another probiotic mixture showed better effectiveness.[31] Ninety-four Danish tourists going on a two-week trip to Egypt were randomized to a mixture of probiotics (*L. acidophilus, L. bulgaricus, Bifidobacterium bifidum,* and *Streptococcus thermophilus*) or a placebo. The dose of probiotic or placebo was started two days prior to travel to allow the probiotic to colonize the intestinal tract, and the treatment was continued until the last day of travel. Significantly fewer tourists given the probiotic mixture developed traveler's diarrhea (43 percent) compared to those given the placebo (71 percent, $p < 0.001$). No adverse reactions were noted during this study.

TREATMENTS FOR TRAVELER'S DIARRHEA

Treatment typically begins after traveler's diarrhea symptoms have occurred, and the treatment strategies vary. Treatment of acute traveler's diarrhea depends on the severity, the person's health, and confidence in self-medication. In one study of 784 tourists, nearly half of whom developed traveler's diarrhea, only 19 (2 percent) sought medical help.[5] The choice to self-medicate may be based on the tourist's belief that traveler's diarrhea usually is not serious and the inconvenience of finding medical care while on vacation is too great. Once traveler's diarrhea develops, the typical treatment for mild traveler's diarrhea may include just waiting it out and drinking more water.

This does nothing to shorten the duration of the diarrhea but will limit dehydration. Treatments for infectious causes of traveler's diarrhea include medications, antibiotics, and probiotics, as no effective vaccines are currently in use to prevent traveler's diarrhea.[6] The advantages and disadvantages of these different treatments are summarized in Table 2.4.

Treatments for traveler's diarrhea:

- *Probiotics*
- *Pepto-Bismol*
- *Antibiotics*

Activated Charcoal

Activated charcoal has been given to patients with traveler's diarrhea, but has not been shown to be effective in controlled trials. Furthermore, charcoal may bind antibiotics or other medications taken at the same time, which interferes with how well the antibiotics work.[35]

TABLE 2.4. Advantages and disadvantages for types of treatments for traveler's diarrhea.

Type of Treatment	Advantages	Disadvantages
Antidiarrheal	Not costly	Many pills per day
Medications	Nonspecific	Not recommended for all Adverse effects common Not for prolonged use
Antibiotic	Good results if pathogen is susceptible	Antibiotic resistance Risk for adverse effects Narrow range of action Can be costly Not for prolonged use
Probiotic	Nonspecific Side effects infrequent Helps host to recover Does not disrupt host systems Inexpensive Good for prolonged use Multiple mechanisms of action	Few large clinical trials have been conducted so exact efficacy is unknown

Medications to Slow Intestinal Motility

Treatment with antidiarrheal medications that act to slow the gut motility, such as loperamide or diphenoxylate, are effective in cases of mild to moderate diarrhea, but need to be combined with an antibiotic when the diarrhea is severe or bloody. These medications should be avoided if the cause is *Salmonella* or *Shigella,* as they tend to prolong the diarrhea.[19,36] Diphenoxylate can have a number of adverse effects, including effects on the central nervous system, urinary retention, constipation, nausea, and ileus (intestinal blockage) and may prevent absorption of nutrients.

Oral Rehydration Solutions

Oral rehydration solutions (ORS) usually are not needed for traveler's diarrhea unless there is severe dehydration or if an infant develops traveler's diarrhea. Different types of rehydration solutions have been shown to be equally effective (intravenous solutions and ORS–low sodium solution).[6] Oral rehydration solutions should not be used in patients with bloody diarrhea, cases of intestinal blockage, or by anyone with mild traveler's diarrhea.

Antibiotic Treatment

Antibiotics used to treat traveler's diarrhea include trimethoprim/sulfamethoxazole (TMP/SMX), doxycycline, rifampin, azithromycin, or fluoroquinolones (for example, ciprofloxacin).[8,20,37] TMP-SMX usually is 70 to 80 percent effective, but resistance to this antibiotic has been steadily increasing worldwide.[19] In Mexico, one study found that TMP/SMX failed to adequately treat 29 percent of tourists with traveler's diarrhea.[38] Ciprofloxacin, which is commonly prescribed to travelers, infrequently causes another form of diarrhea, *Clostridium difficile* disease, so its use is not without risk.[39] In addition, fluoroquinolones are not recommended for children and pregnant women. Ciprofloxacin resistance has been reported in almost all *Campylobacter* strains isolated in military troops with traveler's diarrhea who were serving in Thailand.[18] Rifampin does not work in 9.7 to 11 percent of those with traveler's diarrhea and one of three report adverse effects.[38] A wide range of microorganisms can cause traveler's diarrhea, so the cause may need to be determined before an appropriate antibiotic is given. This is not typically done for traveler's diarrhea unless patients are hospitalized. There is concern about overuse of antibiotics because this leads to antibiotic resistance. Although most antibiotics have a very low rate of serious adverse effects, rare, life-threatening reactions are known to occur. In addition, antibiotics taken to treat traveler's diarrhea may trigger overgrowth syndromes (*Candida* vaginitis or *Clostridium difficile* colitis).

Viral agents such as rotavirus and the Norwalk virus are becoming increasingly common causes of traveler's diarrhea. Specific treatments for viral agents of traveler's diarrhea do not exist, and bismuth subsalicylate treatment is no longer recommended as a treatment for viral causes of traveler's diarrhea.[6] Parasitic infestations may respond to antibiotics such as metronidazole (for *Entamoeba histolytica* and *Giardia lambdia*) or TMP-SMX (for *Cyclospora*).

Antibiotics have a place in the treatment of severe traveler's diarrhea. However, new modalities are needed to treat mild to moderate cases. Unfortunately, few studies have tested probiotics for the treatment of traveler's diarrhea (see Table 2.5). However, the results show promise for this approach.

Saccharomyces boulardii

Two studies were conducted to test if *Saccharomyces boulardii* effectively shortens the duration of traveler's diarrhea. In one study,

TABLE 2.5. Probiotics used for the treatment of traveler's diarrhea.

Probiotic	Population studied	Duration of diarrhea in the probiotic group	Duration of diarrhea in the control group	Reference
Saccharomyces boulardii	60 tourists in Tunisia	2.1 days	1.4 days[*]	Note 40
Saccharomyces boulardii	95 tourists with unresponsive diarrhea	5 days	No control	Note 41

* Probiotic was significantly better than the placebo.

60 tourists with traveler's diarrhea in Tunisia were randomly assigned either *S. boulardii* (600 mg/day) or ethacridine lactate (a typical treatment in Tunisia) for five days.[40] The duration of traveler's diarrhea was significantly longer in the probiotic group (2.1 days, $p =$ 0.04) compared to the standard treatment (1.4 days). Clinically, there is little difference between the durations of diarrhea for these two groups. There were no adverse reactions in the study.

Another study involved 95 patients who had traveler's diarrhea for an average of 11 days and were unresponsive to standard antibiotics. All were treated with *S. boulardii* at a dose of 150 to 450 mg/day (mean of 428 mg/day).[41] The diarrhea stopped in an average of five days. Only 2 of the 95 travelers reported adverse effects. However, no comparison group (untreated) was used in this trial.

Lactobacillus *or Mixtures of Probiotics*

At the time this book went to press, no studies had been published on the treatment of traveler's diarrhea using *Lactobacillus* probiotics or mixtures of probiotics. However, studies show *Lactobacillus* in children with rotavirus infections (one of the causes of acute diarrhea in young children) has been effective in reducing the duration of diarrhea.[42,43] These trials were not conducted with children with traveler's diarrhea. Randomized controlled trials using these *Lactobacillus*-based probiotics for the treatment of traveler's diarrhea may be worthwhile.

Cost-Effectiveness

The most important cost component of traveler's diarrhea is the cost associated with the days of incapacitation. Indirect economic losses incurred by businesses that service travelers are not trivial. Prevention using probiotics is far more cost-effective than treatment using antibiotics. A typical supply of *Lactobacillus* or *Saccharomyces* probiotic averages $15-20.00. In contrast, the average cost of a ten-day course of generic ciprofloxacin (the most widely given antibiotic for traveler's diarrhea) is $80.00.

CONCLUSIONS AND OBSERVATIONS

Use of probiotics to prevent or treat traveler's diarrhea has not been as thoroughly studied as treatments of other types of diarrheal diseases. Scientific proof for the precise effectiveness of probiotics to treat or prevent active traveler's diarrhea is currently lacking. However, the benefits of probiotics in the prevention of traveler's diarrhea appear to be extremely promising. The lack of clinical studies for traveler's diarrhea is surprising, given the frequency of this problem and how disruptive it can be on a trip.

Although there are few studies using probiotics for traveler's diarrhea, the largest market for probiotics in Europe is for the prevention of traveler's diarrhea. The traveler should consider the advantages and disadvantages of each type of therapy when faced with the risk of traveler's diarrhea. Given the recommendations not to use antibiotics or other medications for prevention of traveler's diarrhea, probiotics can offer a safe and effective alternative. As shown in Figure 2.4, the type of probiotic with the highest percent of effective studies is *Saccharomyces boulardii*. Probiotics containing other microbes also may work, but studies to test them have not been reported or were inconclusive.

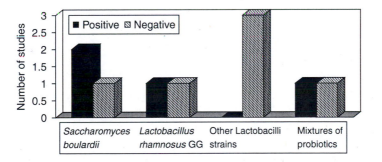

FIGURE 2.4. Number of positive and negative randomized, controlled trials for traveler's diarrhea prevention by different types of probiotics are presented (Positive = effectiveness shown in controlled clinical trial, Negative = no significant effectiveness shown in controlled clinical trial).

Recommendations for Traveler's Diarrhea

- Take probiotics one or two days before trip begins and continue throughout the trip.
- Continue probiotics for one to two days after returning home to allow the body to recover from traveling.
- Continue probiotics for two to four weeks after returning home if you became ill during your trip.
- Use of probiotics for prevention is especially recommended for travelers who have severe intestinal conditions or are immuno-compromised (including HIV) or for those highly susceptible to severe dehydration (the elderly, children, or those with kidney conditions).
- The strongest evidence supports use of *Saccharomyces boulardii* for prevention of traveler's diarrhea.

Chapter 3

Acute Diarrhea

The cause of acute diarrhea is varied and unanticipated. Acute diarrhea strikes the otherwise healthy individual, suddenly and unexpectedly. The episode usually is due to an infectious agent, though most of the time the specific causative microorganism cannot be determined. Situations that place people in developed countries at risk include exposure to schoolchildren or day care centers, hospitalization, being immunocompromised, and improper food handling.

FREQUENTLY ASKED QUESTIONS

Why do more children get diarrhea when they go to day care or begin school?

Children are susceptible to disease-causing organisms, especially to those they have not been exposed to previously. Not only is the child introduced to new sources of infection (for example, other children), but children are in a close environment (for example, an enclosed classroom), which tends to increase the chances of contact with pathogens.

How common is pediatric diarrhea?

In the United States, an estimated 21 to 37 million episodes of diarrhea occur in children every year.

The Power of Probiotics
© 2007 by The Haworth Press, Inc. All rights reserved.
doi:10.1300/5597_03

Are not antibiotics effective against pediatric diarrhea?

Antibiotics have no benefit in 85 to 95 percent of the cases. Most cases of pediatric diarrhea are caused by viruses, which are not susceptible to antibiotics.

Does hand washing help?

Yes, but it is difficult to monitor children all the time to make sure they wash their hands.

Is there anything day care centers and schools can do to reduce the risk?

Yes, they can maintain clean facilities, teach and ensure hand washing, and promote good hygiene. But some of the risk is due to first-time exposures and the crowding together of susceptible children in schools and day care centers.

Do children have a problem taking probiotics?

No, children usually do not have a problem taking probiotics. Children seem to be more open to the idea that they can take "friendly microbes" to help them be healthy. In addition, probiotics can be blended easily into foods that a child likes, such as applesauce.

Are probiotics safe to be given to children?

Probiotics are an attractive alternative to antibiotics, especially for children. Studies conducted with children show that probiotics are well tolerated and have few serious adverse effects. Unlike antibiotics or harsh antidiarrheal medications, which frequently have side effects, probiotics work with the child's natural body defenses to resist disease.

Are probiotics effective against pediatric diarrhea?

Yes, some probiotics have been shown to be effective against pediatric diarrhea.

ACUTE PEDIATRIC DIARRHEA

Pediatric diarrhea is a problem on a global scale. In developed countries, the largest impact is seen when outbreaks of diarrhea sweep through day care centers and preschools in winter. In developing countries, millions of children die every year from pediatric diarrhea. As most cases of pediatric diarrhea are due to viruses, there are no effective antibiotics for these infections. Probiotics are effective for the prevention and treatment of this type of illness and are well tolerated by children.

Epidemiology of Pediatric Diarrhea

Diarrhea is common among children, and the consequences of a severe case of acute pediatric diarrhea can be serious. In the United States, 16.5 million children below the age of five years have at least one episode of diarrhea a year.[1] Pediatric diarrhea also places a heavy burden on the U.S. health care system: Three million physician visits and 163,000 hospitalizations occur per year (13 percent of all hospital visits for children younger than five years are due to pediatric diarrhea). In developing countries, 3.2 million children die every year due to diarrhea, and this can account for as much as 25 percent of their national health care costs.[2] The prevalence of pediatric diarrhea depends upon the age of the child. Neonates (birth to one month) have high frequencies (up to 64 percent).[3] For young infants (< 2 years old), the frequency ranges from 3 to 50 percent; and for older children (3 to 18 years), the frequency is 5 to 8 percent, which is similar to adult frequencies. There also may be an increased frequency when children are in day care centers.

Children are prone to intestinal disorders because their gastrointestinal tracts are developing and maturing, and they do not frequently wash their hands. Their bodies are not as resilient as those of adults are in combating diseases. Children also are exposed for the first time to many of the causes (bacteria or viruses) and are placed in settings that put them at higher risk for exposure (day care centers, nurseries, schools, etc.). As the child is exposed to specific organisms that cause disease, antibodies are produced and the body develops a memory of those pathogenic organisms so that future exposures result in faster production of protective antibodies at higher concentrations than the first exposure. However, children do not develop this immune memory for all the pathogens they will be exposed to during their development (see Figure 3.1 for sizes of different pathogens).

A common symptom of many pediatric diseases is diarrhea, and in these cases the diarrhea may not be due to the presence of a pathogen. In developing countries, poor nutrition results in a weakened immune system. Both the weakened immune system and the increased exposure to pathogens due to poor hygiene and inadequate sanitation may help explain why more children die of pediatric diarrhea in these countries than those in developed countries.

Common Causes of Acute Pediatric Diarrhea

Bacteria	Viruses	Parasites
Salmonella	Rotavirus	Giardia lambdia
Shigella	Adenovirus	Amoebic organisms
Escherichia coli (E. coli)		
Campylobacter		
Clostridium difficile		
Yersinia		

There are many causes of pediatric diarrhea. Bacteria and viruses (see preceding table) are common causes of diarrhea in children. Other causes, such as lactose intolerance or other types of food allergies also are common. Outbreaks of pediatric diarrhea can be due to food poisoning (usually *Salmonella* and, less commonly, *Shigella* or *E. coli*).

Outbreaks of pediatric diarrhea occur in hospitals, and may be caused by a bacterium called *Clostridium difficile* or a virus called rotavirus.[3] During the first few weeks of life, as many as 64 percent of infants become colonized with *C. difficile* if they are delivered in the hospital, but usually do not develop diarrhea as a result.[3] Older children and adults usually are protected from *C. difficile* because normal intestinal microflora inhibit the overgrowth of this pathogen by a phenomenon called "colonization resistance" (see Chapter 1).[4] *C. difficile* disease usually does not occur in adults unless antibiotics or other

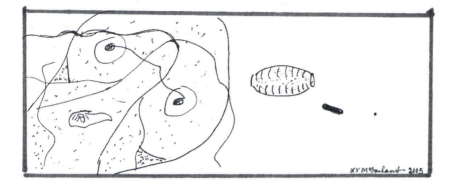

FIGURE 3.1. Relative size of pathogens for pediatric diarrhea. From left to right: the top part of a trophozoite of parasite called *Giardia lambdia* (8,000 times larger than a bacterium); a yeast (15 times larger than a bacterium); a bacterium, such as *Escherichia coli* and representation of a rotavirus (100 to 1000 times smaller than a bacterium). *Source:* Illustration by Lynne V. McFarland.

factors disrupt this colonization resistance. However, since the neonatal intestine is immature and lacks the protective normal microflora established in adults, children are susceptible to bacterial colonization and overgrowth. The source of *C. difficile* usually is not the mother but is exposure to *C. difficile* spores in the hospital nursery.[5] Researchers found that 60 percent of neonates in a hospital nursery were colonized by *C. difficile,* and 50 percent of the environmental surfaces tested positive for *C. difficile* spores.[6] Another study followed up 451 newborns in five postnatal wards in England.[7] In total, 65 of 451 (14.4 percent) neonates were positive for *C. difficile.* More than half of the 32 infants in one ward tested positive. Other outbreaks among children have been reported in pediatric oncology wards, pediatric orthopedic services, neonatal wards, and day care centers.[3] Despite the high presence of *C. difficile,* the frequency of diarrheal symptoms in neonatal outbreaks usually is only 5 to 8 percent.[3]

Viral causes of pediatric diarrhea commonly are rotavirus infections. These infections occur most often during winter in schools, day care centers, and hospital pediatric wards. Outbreaks of rotaviral infections are common. These viruses can remain alive on hands or inanimate surfaces for many days, and spread easily by casual contact via the fecal-oral route. Rotaviral infections do not respond to antibiotics, and an early vaccine with the potential to protect children from developing rotaviral infections had problems in development. The vaccine being tested was withdrawn from clinical trials because of intussusception (enfolding of one segment of the intestine within another). A new vaccine has now been approved. Based on one large study, the new vaccine does not appear to have the risk for intussusception. The need for a safe and effective treatment and prevention modality for rotaviral infections is apparent.

The consequences of pediatric diarrhea range from mild to severe. Sometimes, the diarrhea is self-limited (the body cures itself with no treatment). Other times, hospitalization may be required. Children are especially prone to severe dehydration, which can be life threatening, and may develop within just a few days. Therefore, it is important to keep track of a child with diarrhea and seek professional help if symptoms worsen. Treatment should be considered if the diarrhea is prolonged over two days, if fever develops, or if the child is lethargic. The diarrhea also may progress into colitis, which is diarrhea with inflammation of the large bowel. Infrequently, pediatric colitis may progress to pseudomembranous colitis, toxic megacolon (an extremely dilated colon), or other types of inflammatory colitis. Symptoms of colitis may include profuse watery diarrhea, intense abdominal pain, hyperthermia (unusually high fever), edema (swelling), and painful ascites (fluid in the abdominal cavity). Pseudomembranous colitis is an inflammatory type of colitis, characterized by an inner membrane that coats the inside of the intestine. It is caused by *C. difficile,* which can overgrow when antibiotics are used. The most commonly implicated antibiotics causing *C. difficile* colitis in children are similar to those involved in adult cases (penicillins, cephalosporins, or lincosamides). Although pseudomembranous colitis is rare, the consequences may be severe. A study found that nearly one in four children with pediatric pseudomembranous colitis dies.[8] One researcher also described seven cases of fatal pseudomembranous colitis in children aged 13 days to 17 years.[9] Children also may develop recurrent *C. difficile* disease (repeated episodes of diarrhea, which may extend over several years); recurrence rates from 15 to 57 percent have been reported, even after treatment with standard antibiotics targeted against *C. difficile.*[3]

Children with cystic fibrosis are also at risk for *C. difficile* infection, most likely because of the regular use of antibiotics. In fact, about 50 percent of children with cystic fibrosis harbor *C. difficile,* but fortunately this colonization only occasionally results in diarrhea or pseudomembranous colitis.

Necrotizing enterocolitis is the most common intestinal catastrophe in premature neonates, and it is thought to be caused by overgrowth of pathogenic bacteria after enteral (tube) feedings and interruption of blood flow to the intestine. Fortunately, the frequency is low (1 to 3 cases per 1,000 live births) unless the birth weight is below 1,500 g, when the frequency reaches 7 percent.[10] Mortality in the very low birth weight neonates because of necrotizing enterocolitis can be quite high (50 percent). Premature formula-fed babies are at the highest risk. Babies who are breast-fed have a lower risk of this condition, which may be due to the presence of higher levels of bifidobacteria, a type of protective bacteria that resists the growth of pathogenic organisms.

Treatments for Pediatric Diarrhea

Self-Limiting Diarrhea

Usually, the child does not require specific treatment and the diarrhea resolves spontaneously. Unfortunately, it is impossible to predict whether a child will recover spontaneously or go on to develop serious diarrheal disease or other complications. If the diarrhea seems to be associated with antibiotic use, it may be possible to stop the diarrhea by simply discontinuing the antibiotic, but only if medically reasonable. However, most cases of pediatric diarrhea are not associated with antibiotic use.

Antibiotics

If the cause of the diarrhea is a bacterium susceptible to antibiotic treatment, an appropriate antibiotic can be effective. However, since most (85 to 95 percent) pediatric diarrhea is due to viral infections, antibiotics provide no benefits in a majority of the cases. If the cause is *C. difficile,* treatment with metronidazole or vancomycin may be started. Metronidazole is associated with a higher frequency of side effects, including nausea, metallic taste, vomiting, numbness in toes and fingers, and, rarely, convulsions. Concerns with the expense of vancomycin and the increasing frequency of vancomycin-resistant bacteria have limited its use. There are no clear treatment recommendations for infants and children infected with *C. difficile*. Vancomycin usually is given for only severe cases of pseudomembranous colitis, recurrent colitis, or to children with compromised immune systems. Recurrences of *C. difficile* have been noted in several studies; the frequency ranges from 43 to 67 percent after vancomycin is discontinued.[3]

Antibiotic treatment may not be appropriate for other causes of pediatric diarrhea. Antibiotics have no effect on viruses, so diarrhea caused by viruses (such as rotavirus) should not be treated with antibiotics. Antibiotic treatments are inappropriate for other causes of bacterial diarrhea as antibiotics have been shown to extend the length of time children carry the organism (for example, *Salmonella* infections).

Oral Rehydration Therapy

Dehydration is a serious problem for children who develop diarrhea, and may lead to hospitalization or death. Because most cases of pediatric diarrhea do not respond to antibiotics, an appropriate therapy is to treat dehydration by providing liquids and replacing electrolytes. This is called oral rehydration therapy. Although this treats one of the more serious symptoms of pediatric diarrhea, it does nothing to eliminate the pathogen causing the diarrhea or to restore the child's intestinal health and microbial balance.

Probiotic Treatments

Much research has tested various types of probiotics for the treatment of pediatric diarrhea. It is critical to be both protective and cautious with medications for children. An important research goal is to find treatments that are effective without causing undue stress or complications to the vulnerable child's body. Antibiotics often are too harsh and may be ineffective for children with diarrhea. On the other hand, some probiotics have been found to be both effective and well tolerated by children.

Saccharomyces boulardii. Many studies support the use of *S. boulardii* for treatment of childhood diarrhea (see Table 3.1). Three clinical trials compared the effectiveness of *S. boulardii,* with a placebo control group, and all three found that the probiotic was effective.[11-13] The largest study involved 130 children (aged three months to three years) with acute diarrhea who were receiving oral rehydration therapy.[11] The children were randomly assigned for a four-day treatment with either *S. boulardii* (200 mg every eight hours) or placebo (glucose solution). More of the children (85 percent) treated with *S. boulardii* experienced a reduction of diarrhea compared to only 40 percent of the placebo group. In another study, 38 infants hospitalized with acute diarrhea and receiving oral rehydration therapy were divided into two groups.[12] *Saccharomyces boulardii* was given to half the children at a dose of 500 mg per day for five days, while the other half who did not receive the probiotic acted as controls. The children treated with the probiotic had significant reductions in both the number of stools per day and the time it took for the diar-

TABLE 3.1. Clinical trials of single probiotics for treatment of pediatric diarrhea.

Probiotic	Age of subjects (months)	Number in the study	Dose given per day	Duration of treatment (days)	Percentage cured or duration of diarrhea (days) in the probiotic group versus controls	Reference
Saccharomyces boulardii	3-36	130	2×10^{10}	4	85* versus 40	Note 11
Saccharomyces boulardii	0.5-30	38	1×10^{10}	5	95* versus 79	Note 12
Saccharomyces boulardii	11-35	18	Varied	30	59* versus. 24	Note 13
Lactobacillus acidophilus LB (killed strain)	Not given	103	varied	Not given	1.0 versus 1.1 ns	Note 14
Lactobacillus acidophilus (killed strain)	3-24	73	2×10^{10}	3	1.8 versus 2.4 ns	Note 15
Lactobacillus reuteri	3-36	40	10^{10}-10^{11}	5	1.7 versus 2.9 ns	Note 16
Lactobacillus reuteri	6-36	66	10^{10}-10^{11}	5	1.5* versus 2.5	Note 17
Lactobacillus casei DN	7-32	287	2×10^{10}	90	4.3* versus 8.0	Note 18

*Probiotic was significantly more effective than controls ($p < 0.05$).

ns = not significant.

rhea to stop. Most of the children (95 percent) were cured if *S. boulardii* was given along with rehydration, while 79 percent treated with only oral rehydration were cured. Other researchers tested *S. boulardii* in a double-blinded trial of "toddler diarrhea" and found that 59 percent improved after one month if given *S. boulardii*, compared to only 24 percent children given placebo.[13] No significant adverse effects were reported in the three studies.

Sometimes it is possible to study a group of children who all have the same cause of diarrhea. A French scientist studied 19 children (ages 2-32 months, median of 8 months) with chronic diarrhea (lasting over 15 days) caused by *C. difficile*.[19] *S. boulardii* was given orally for 15 days, according to the age of the child (500 mg/day for < 1-year-olds, 750 mg/day for 1- to 4-year-olds and 1 g/day for > 4-year-olds). No antibiotics were given during the treatment part of the trial. Within one week, symptoms resolved in 18 of the 19 children. No side effects were noted. Two children had a subsequent relapse of disease, which resolved rapidly after a second treatment with *S. boulardii*. As this study did not have a control group, it is uncertain as to how many of the children would have recovered eventually with no probiotic treatment, but the results are promising for this very persistent and serious form of childhood diarrhea.

Lactobacillus preparations. Several types of *Lactobacillus* probiotics have been shown to be effective treatments for pediatric diarrhea (see Table 3.2). A review of nine children's studies that involved children treated with a *Lactobacillus* probiotic (either *L. rhamnosus, L. acidophilus, L. reuteri,* or a mix of different lactobacilli probiotics) and a group receiving no probiotic treatment concluded that *Lactobacillus* treatments were effective for pediatric diarrhea.[1,15-17,21,25,28-30,32] Although the effect of the *Lactobacillus* treatment was mild (most studies usually report a one-day reduction of the duration of diarrhea), higher doses of lactobacilli appeared to be more beneficial. In the nine reviewed studies, *Lactobacillus* probiotics remained effective, regardless of the cause of diarrhea (rotavirus or some pathogens), or geographic location. These studies also found a similar frequency of adverse effects in the probiotics-treated children, as was observed in the control children.[16,28]

Studies not included in that review have tested other strains of lactobacilli for the treatment of pediatric diarrhea (see Table 3.1).

TABLE 3.2. Clinical trials of *Lactobacillus rhamnosus* GG for treatment of pediatric diarrhea.

Age of subjects (months)	Number in the study	Dose given per day	Duration of treatment (days)	Percent cured or days of diarrhea in the probiotic group compared to controls	Reference
<24	124	1×10^6	7	1.6 versus 1.6 ns	Note 20
1-36	287	4×10^{10}	Varied	2.4* versus 3.0	Note 21
3-36	100	Not given	2	1.9* versus 3.3	Note 22
4-45	71	2×10^{10}-10^{11}	5	1.4* versus 2.4	Note 23
5-28	42	2×10^{10}	5	1.5* versus 2.3	Note 24
7-37	39	2×10^{10}-10^{11}	5	1.1* versus 2.5	Note 25
6-35	49	Not given	5	1.8* versus 2.8	Note 26
<24	39	Not given	2	1.9 versus 3.3 ns	Note 27
1-24	32	2×10^{10}-10^{11}	2	69* versus 25	Note 28
1-36	123	5×10^9	5	2.7* versus 3.8	Note 29

*Probiotic was significantly more effective than controls ($p < 0.05$).

ns = not significant; *Lactobacillus* GG = *Lactobacillus rhamnosus.* GG

One looked at 287 children aged 7 to 32 months old with acute diarrhea.[18] The children treated with *Lactobacillus casei*-fermented milk had a shorter duration of diarrhea (4.3 days) compared to children given control milk (8.0 days, $p = 0.009$).

Two studies that used a killed preparation of a *Lactobacillus* probiotic did not find a large difference between the probiotics-treated group and the control group with no probiotics, indicating the probiotic needs to be living to be effective.[14,15] The two studies that tested the same probiotic, *Lactobacillus reuteri,* are interesting because one found a significant effect[17] and the other did not[16] (see Table 3.1). In the study that found a significant decrease in diarrhea,[17] the children were treated with a slightly higher probiotic dose and for an additional two days. Interestingly, the probiotic was effective in only the children with rotavirus infections and not the children with mixed causes of diarrhea.

Lactobacillus GG (also known as *Lactobacillus rhamnosus* GG) is the single most studied *Lactobacillus* strain for pediatric diarrhea (Table 3.2). Over 800 children have been enrolled in ten controlled clinical trials studying *Lactobacillus* GG for the treatment of pediatric diarrhea. Eight of these trials found that the probiotic shortened the duration of the diarrhea. One hundred Italian children who had mild rotaviral diarrhea were enrolled in one study.[22] They were given either *Lactobacillus* GG with oral rehydration or received oral rehydration alone for two days. The duration of diarrhea in the control group averaged three days, while the children given *Lactobacillus* GG had a significantly shorter duration of diarrhea (an average of two days, $p < 0.05$). In addition, far fewer children who received the probiotic were shedding rotavirus at the end of two days (12.9 percent) compared to children who did not receive the probiotic (83.3 percent). Reducing the time for children to shed rotavirus limits the spread of infections to other children. A large clinical trial was conducted in ten countries to test *Lactobacillus* GG with oral rehydration versus placebo with oral rehydration in children aged one month to three years with acute diarrhea.[21] The most common causes were rotavirus (35 percent) and bacterial (18 percent). Children treated with *Lactobacillus* GG had significantly shorter duration of diarrhea (2.4 days) compared to 3.0 days in controls ($p < 0.03$). Another important finding was a significantly shorter hospitalization for the *Lactobacillus*-GG-treated children (an average of 79 hours) compared to the control children (an average of 96 hours, $p = 0.04$). Getting children out of the hospital and back home is an important objective for both the family and health care providers, and reduces health care costs associated with pediatric diarrhea. A study in Brazil examined 124 male children under the age of two years who had severe diarrhea.[20] Oral rehydration solution was given to all the children. They then were given either *Lactobacillus* GG or placebo capsules for seven days. In this group of children with severe diarrhea (about 50 percent were caused by rotaviral infections), the lactobacillus probiotic provided no apparent benefits. The diarrhea resolved quickly in both groups (1.6 days). The authors concluded that in this situation the diarrhea resolved too quickly for the probiotic to be effective in either group.

Lactobacillus GG has been used to successfully treat other cases of pediatric rotaviral diarrhea. A study in Finland involved 71 well-nourished children between 4 and 45 months of age, who were having acute diarrhea (82 percent cause by rotavirus).[23] The children were randomly assigned to one of three groups: *Lactobacillus* GG

(125 mg, twice a day for five days) in a milk product, *Lactobacillus* GG (125 mg, twice a day for five days) in capsule form, or placebo (125 mg, twice a day for five days) in yogurt. The vehicle of delivery (milk product or capsule) did not affect the treatment outcome, as the diarrhea lasted an average of 1.4 days in both *Lactobacillus* GG groups. The children treated with the placebo yogurt had significantly longer duration of diarrhea (mean of 2.4 days, $p < 0.001$). The effectiveness of *Lactobacillus* GG on rotaviral diarrhea was confirmed in a second study with 42 children aged 5 to 28 months, all of whom had rotaviral diarrhea.[24] The children were randomly assigned to either *Lactobacillus* GG (given as a freeze-dried powder in capsules at 125 mg, twice daily for five days) or placebo. Once again, the duration of diarrhea was significantly shorter in children treated with *Lactobacillus* GG (an average of 1.5 days) than in children given placebo (an average of 2.3 days, $p = 0.002$). A third study of 39 children with rotaviral infections also found a shorter duration of diarrhea in *Lactobacillus*-GG-treated children (mean of 1.1 days) compared to children given placebo (mean of 2.5 days, $p = 0.001$).[25] The same study also tried to determine why *Lactobacillus* GG was beneficial against rotaviral infections by looking at the effect of the probiotic on the immune response to rotaviral exposure. Of the *Lactobacillus*-GG-treated children, 90 percent developed IgA-specific (protective) antibodies against rotavirus by the end of the five days of treatment compared to only 46 percent of the placebo group ($p = 0.006$). Stimulation of the immune system to produce antibodies that kill rotavirus is a likely explanation for how some probiotics work against this pathogen. Not all probiotic strains can stimulate protective antibodies. In another study, children with rotaviral infections were given either *Lactobacillus* GG, *Lactobacillus casei,* or a mixture (*Streptococcus thermophilus* and *Lactobacillus delbruckii* subspecies *bulgaricus*) for five days.[26] Only the children given *Lactobacillus* GG showed a significant rise in IgA antibodies protective against rotavirus. Later studies showed that living *Lactobacillus* GG produced higher levels of protective antibodies against rotavirus than do killed preparations.[32]

No randomized controlled clinical trials for the treatment of *C. difficile* disease in children using *Lactobacillus* GG have been reported at the time this book went to press. Promising results were seen in a case-series report of four children (aged 5 to 70 months, mean 34 months) with a history of recurrent *C. difficile*.[33] *Lactobacillus* GG was given to all four children for two weeks at a dose of 125 mg twice a day. No antibiotics (vancomycin or metronidazole) were given during the treatment part of the trial, but all patients took antibiotics in the follow-up period (median of 9.5 months). All four children responded clinically within five to seven days and were symptom-free by the end of the two-week treatment. No adverse effects were noted. Two (50 percent) of the children had relapses within two months after *Lactobacillus* GG was discontinued.

Mixtures of probiotics. Five large clinical trials with control groups have tested mixtures of probiotics, but only two showed significant effectiveness (see Table 3.3). A study involving 100 children aged 6

TABLE 3.3. Clinical trials of mixtures of probiotics for treatment of pediatric diarrhea.

Probiotic Mix	Age of subjects (months)	Number in the study	Dose given per day	Duration of treatment (days)	Days of diarrhea in the probiotic group compared to controls*	Reference
L. acidophilus, L. bulgaricus and Strept lactis	2-36	54	2×10^9	3	2.5 versus 2.8 ns	Note 30
L. acidophilus and Bifido-bacterium infantis	6-60	100	6×10^9	4	3.1* versus 3.6	Note 34
L. acidophilus and L. bulgaricus and Strept. thermophilus	<36	94	$4\text{-}8 \times 10^8$	Varied	2.7 versus 2.1 ns	Note 31
Lactobacillus rhamnosus 19070-2 and L. reuteri DSM	6-36	69	4×10^{10}	5	3.4 versus 4.2 ns	Note 35
Lactobacillus rhamnosus 19070-2 and L. reuteri DSM	9-44	43	4×10^{10}	5	3.2* versus 4.8	Note 36

*Probiotic was significantly more effective than controls ($p < 0.05$).

to 60 months who had acute diarrhea randomized them to either a probiotic mixture of *Lactobacillus acidophilus* and *Bifidobacterium infantis* or a control group that received only oral rehydration.[31] This probiotic mixture was given for 4 days and significantly reduced the duration of acute diarrhea (3.1 days) compared to the control group (3.6 days, $p < 0.01$). Another group of researchers studied 69 hospitalized children aged 6 to 36 months with acute diarrhea and randomized them to either placebo or a mix of probiotic strains (*Lactobacillus rhamnosus* 19070-2 and *Lactobacillus reuteri* DSM 12246) for five days.[33] Although the duration of diarrhea was reduced in the children given the probiotic mixture (3.4 days), it was not significantly reduced compared to those given placebo (4.2 days). Comparing the two studies in this section shows the impact the number of participants in a study has on the interpretation of the outcome. Smaller differences in a larger study may be statistically significant, whereas a larger difference in a smaller study may not be significant. However, by the end of the treatment phase, only 10 percent of those given the probiotic mixture still experienced diarrhea, whereas 33 percent of the children in the control group had persistent diarrhea ($p = 0.02$). This study illustrates the complexity of evaluating the conclusions of clinical studies. The result may depend on what outcome is evaluated. The study discussed hereafter shows that the subjects studied can strongly influence the outcome.

The same group of researchers did another study with the same probiotic mixture, but instead of looking at children who were hospitalized, they chose nonhospitalized children attending day care centers.[34] These children were not as ill as were the hospitalized children in the first study. The effect of the probiotic mixture was more pronounced, and the children treated with it had a significantly shorter duration of diarrhea (3.2 days) compared to the control group (4.8 days, $p = 0.05$). Three other studies testing different probiotic mixtures did not show a significant probiotic treatment effect (Table 3.3).

Prevention of Pediatric Diarrhea

It is always better to prevent disease from starting than trying to treat disease that has become established and has caused damage to the host. To this end, the proven practices of frequent hand washing, use of clean water, hygienic food preparation, and excellent sanitation will go far in reducing the risk of pediatric diarrhea. Probiotics also can play a preventative role. Probiotics lend themselves uniquely to prophylaxis as their mechanisms of action involve strengthening the normal microbial flora already present in a healthy person and boosting the immune response to potential pathogenic organisms. Prevention also is a valuable strategy in countries with limited resources (prevention of disease reduces the need for hospitalization, medication, and physician visits) or for particularly susceptible populations (undernourished children, ill elderly, and those with chronic conditions). Seven large controlled trials showed various probiotics were significantly effective in preventing pediatric diarrhea in a variety of settings (see Table 3.4). A study of undernourished children in Peru tested whether *Lactobacillus* GG could decrease the risk of childhood diarrhea in the developing country.[43] In this study, 204 healthy children aged 6-24 months were randomized to either *Lactobacillus* GG or placebo for 15 months. At the end of the study, the frequency of diarrhea was significantly less for the *Lactobacillus* GG group (5.2 episodes per child per year) than the children receiving placebo (6.0 episodes per child per year, $p = 0.03$).

Another study found that a probiotic containing both *Lactobacillus acidophilus* and *Bifidobacterium infantis* was effective in preventing cases of necrotizing enterocolitis in newborns.[42] At a neonatal intensive care unit in Bogota, Columbia, 1,237 children were given this probiotic mixture at 5×10^6 cfu/day for the duration of their hospital stay. The incidence of necrotizing enterocolitis in this group was significantly lower (2.7 percent) than the incidence in a control group (6.6 percent, $p < 0.005$) of 1,282 children at the same hospital during the previous year. This result is promising, but needs to be confirmed by another study that is randomized and tests both groups simultaneously. The use of probiotics for necrotizing enterocolitis is an example of a probiotic preventing a life-threatening disease.

Probiotics can be given in a familiar food product that children like to eat or drink instead of in capsules. In France, 928 healthy children were fed either milk fermented by yogurt cultures (control) or milk fermented with probiotic *Lactobacillus casei* strain DN114. The children were followed-up for two months to see if they developed diarrhea.[38] Of the children who drank the *Lactobacillus casei* DN114 milk,

TABLE 3.4. Clinical trials of probiotics for prevention of pediatric diarrhea.

Probiotic Mix	Age of subjects (months)	Number in the study	Dose given per day	Duration of treatment (days)	Incidence of diarrhea in the probiotic group compared to controls*	Reference
Lactobacillus reuteri	12-36	243	10^6-10^{10}	98	24%* versus 36%	Note 37
Lactobacillus casei DN114	6-24	928	1×10^{10}	60	15.9%* versus 22%	Note 38
Lactobacillus GG	1-36	81	1.2×10^{10}	Varied	6.7%* versus 33%	Note 39
Lactobacillus GG	6-120	188	2×10^{10}	10	7%* versus 26%	Note 40
Bifidobacterium bifidum and *Strept. thermophilus*	5-24	55	2×10^8	Varied	7%* versus 31%	Note 41
Lactobacillus acidophilus and *Bifidobacterium infantis*	<1	2519	5×10^7	Varied	2.7%* versus 6.6%	Note 42
Lactobacillus GG	18-29	204	4×10^{10}	450	5.2* versus 6.0**	Note 43

*Probiotic was significantly more effective than controls, $p < 0.05$.

**Episodes of diarrhea per child per year, $p = 0.03$.

Lactobacillus GG = *Lactobacillus rhamnosus* GG.

only 15.9 percent developed diarrhea, compared to significantly more (22 percent) of those drinking the control milk.

Probiotics given as a preventive measure may reduce the number of new cases of pediatric diarrhea using several mechanisms:

- Boosting the immune response
- Shielding the intestinal attachment sites from invading pathogens
- Producing substances that combat the pathogen
- Directly affecting the pathogen itself

Probiotics may reduce the number of viruses that a child sheds into the environment, thereby reducing the risk of infecting others. Researchers in Baltimore, Maryland, gave 55 hospitalized children either nonsupplemented infant formula (controls) or infant formula supplemented with a mix of *Bifidobacterium bifidum* and *Streptococcus thermophilus*.[41] Not only did fewer children who were given the probiotic mixture develop diarrhea (7 percent compared to 31 percent of controls), fewer of the children given the probiotic mixture shed rotavirus during their hospitalization (only 10 percent compared to 39 percent of the controls, $p = 0.02$). This is a valuable way to reduce the incidence of outbreaks of rotaviral diarrhea, which are common in hospitals and day care facilities.

Conclusions and Observations for Pediatric Diarrhea

In the numerous clinical trials discussed in this section, nearly three-quarters showed a significantly beneficial effect of the probiotic. Probiotics given to prevent disease have the strongest therapeutic effect on children (100 percent of preventive trials showed a significant benefit of the probiotic). In contrast, probiotics given to treat an already established disease were effective in 65 percent of the studies. Positive studies showed a decrease in duration of diarrhea of one to two days. While this effect may seem small, caregivers and parents realize that reducing diarrhea by even a day or two is beneficial. Furthermore, prolonged diarrhea can lead to dehydration, electrolyte imbalance, and other complications.

There are several reasons why probiotics may work better in some situations of pediatric diarrhea than others. Selection of an appropriate probiotic strain was shown to be important; more research needs to be done to determine the best strains to use in probiotic mixtures. Probiotics also work better in some populations than others. Probiotic treatment of existing diarrhea appears to be more effective for nonhospitalized children. Probiotics are especially useful in treating and preventing diarrhea caused by rotavirus. None of these studies reported any serious side effects of the probiotic treatment, showing that probiotics are well tolerated by children. Probiotics may offer a viable treatment for children with diarrhea because the organisms work with the natural body systems and microflora, do not traumatize the child's normal functioning, are inexpensive, and are well tolerated.

Recommendations for Pediatric Diarrhea

- For the treatment of diarrhea: Give one to three capsules per day of probiotic while the child has diarrhea and continue for one to two days afterward. If fever or severe diarrhea develops, seek medical attention.
- Prevention of diarrhea: Give one to three capsules per day of probiotic during the period of time when the child is in a high-risk environment, such as a hospital or underdeveloped country.
- Probiotics with the most evidence for benefit are *Lactobacillus rhamnosus* GG and *Saccharomyces boulardii*.

ACUTE ADULT DIARRHEA

Frequently Asked Questions

Why does acute adult diarrhea receive little media attention?

Most cases of adult diarrhea are associated with travel or antibiotic use. Traveler's diarrhea and antibiotics-associated diarrhea are topics covered in Chapters 2 and 4. Most cases of acute adult diarrhea are sporadic (that is, they occur in one person at a time), hence they do not create the kind of interest seen when a pediatric or cruise ship outbreak occurs.

How is acute adult diarrhea different from pediatric diarrhea?

Acute adult diarrhea, not associated with travel or antibiotic use, is less common than pediatric diarrhea and rarely involves rotaviruses. Pediatric diarrhea is very common and usually involves rotaviruses.

Are probiotics helpful in cases of acute adult diarrhea?

There are only a few studies, but probiotics seem helpful.

Here we discuss acute adult diarrhea not associated with travel (see Chapter 2) or antibiotic use (see Chapter 4). Acute adult diarrhea is a broad classification for diarrhea that includes illnesses that may develop quickly but are short-lived and occur in individuals, not in outbreaks. Most experience occasional episodes of acute diarrhea of unknown origin. The difficulty in treating adults with "acute diarrhea" is that there are so many different causes. In contrast, pediatric diarrhea is mostly due to rotavirus. Some adult diarrheas have a bacterial origin involving well-known pathogens such as salmonella, campylobacter, *Vibrio cholerae,* or enterotoxigenic *Escherichia coli,* or involve parasites such as *Entamoeba histolytica.* However, the vast majority are of unknown origin. The impact of cholera is extremely important in underdeveloped countries; an effective, inexpensive, and practical treatment as an alternative to antibiotics would be of great benefit. The other causes of adult diarrhea result in less dramatic infections but impact the health care system and disrupt the daily lives of working adults. Only two probiotics, *Enterococcus faecium* strain SF68 and *Saccharomyces boulardii,* have been tested and the results reported for acute adult diarrhea (see Table 3.5).

Most acute adult diarrhea episodes last only one to two days, and do not require treatment

Probiotic Treatment of Adult Diarrhea

Enterococcus faecium *SF68*

Three large studies have tested the effectiveness of this probiotic for adults with acute diarrhea. Patients with acute diarrhea, who were enrolled in two hospitals in Belgium, took part in one study.[44] 185 adults were randomly given either *Enterococcus faecium* SF68 or placebo for five days. When tested for the cause of their diarrhea, 14 percent were due to *Salmonella* or *Campylobacter* infections, but the rest of the cases did not have an identifiable cause. Even though the types of diarrhea were diverse, patients given the *Enterococcus faecium* SF68 had a shorter duration of diarrhea (1.7 days) than those given placebo (2.8 days). This finding was confirmed in a study of 78 Swiss patients, of whom 92 percent of those treated with *Enterococcus faecium* SF68 were cured in seven days, compared to 87 percent of those given placebo.[46] However, this probiotic was not found to be effective in very serious forms of diarrhea: cholera and entero-

TABLE 3.5. Probiotics for the treatment of acute adult diarrhea.

Probiotic	Study population	Probiotic treatment	Effect in the probiotic group*	Effect in the control group	Reference
Enterococcus faecium SF68	185 adults with diarrhea in Belgium	4.5×10^8/ day for 5 days	1.7 ± 0.6 days[¶]	2.8 ± 0.9 days	Note 44
Enterococcus faecium SF68	183 adults in Bangladesh with either cholera or *E. Coli* diarrhea	4×10^9/ day for 3 days	3 days (cholera) and 1 day (*E. coli*) ns	3 days (cholera) and 1 day (*E. coli*)	Note 45
Enterococcus faecium SF68	78 Swiss adults with acute diarrhea	2.2×10^8/ day for 7 days	92.5%[¶]	86.8%	Note 46
S. boulardii	92 German outpatient adults with acute diarrhea	300-600 mg/day for 8 days	-17.2[¶,†]	-13.6	Note 47
S. boulardii	35 French AIDS patients with chronic diarrhea	3 g/day for 7 days	61%[¶]	12%	Note 48
S. boulardii	11 American HIV+ patients with chronic diarrhea	2-3 g/day for 14 days	6/11 cured	No control	Note 49
S. boulardii	54 adults with *E.* histolytic amoebic dysentery	750 mg/day for 10 days	100% cure[¶]	82%	Note 50

*Outcomes are duration of diarrhea in days, or percent cured of diarrhea by end of study, or diarrhea score.

[¶]Probiotic significantly more effective than controls, $p < 0.05$.

ns = not significant.

[†]Diarrhea score based on stool frequency and consistency (lower the score, the less the diarrhea). A score of -17.2 indicates less diarrhea than a score of -13.6.

toxigenic *E. coli*. The duration of diarrhea was the same in 183 adults in Bangladesh who had either cholera or *E. coli* infections, irrespective of whether they were given *Enterococcus faecium* SF68 or placebo.[45] This study is of limited value, however, because the patients were treated for only three days. The results of this study do not prove that probiotics are ineffective for cholera or *E. coli* infections as the diarrhea persisted past the short time of treatment.

Saccharomyces boulardii

This yeast probiotic showed promise in a study of 92 outpatient adults with acute diarrhea,[47] but no other studies have been conducted to confirm this finding (Table 3.5). *S. boulardii* may be effective in controlling chronic diarrhea associated with advanced AIDS. Two studies tested *S. boulardii* in patients with advanced HIV infections. In France, 35 AIDS patients with chronic diarrhea were given either *S. boulardii* or placebo for seven days. At the end of the study, 61 percent of those given the probiotic were cured while significantly fewer of those given placebo (12 percent) responded.[48] The dose of *S. boulardii* was higher (3 g/day) than that usually given in other studies, but there were no reported side effects of this high dose in these extremely ill patients. Another study also found that at least 2 to 3 g of *S. boulardii* per day is needed to show a significant decrease in diarrhea among HIV-positive patients.[49] Considering that AIDS is a global problem and there are no effective, inexpensive, and practical treatments for the debilitating chronic diarrhea that afflicts these patients, more studies of probiotics with HIV-positive patients should be carried out to define the effectiveness of the probiotic approach.

S. boulardii was shown to have efficacy in the treatment of amoebic dysentery (diarrhea with bloody stools due to infection by protozoa). Adults infected with *Entamoeba histolytica* in Iran were given standard therapy (metronidazole and iodoqinol) and half of them also were given *S. boulardii*. Adults given the yeast probiotic were cured more rapidly (average of 12 hours until symptoms of dysentery stopped) compared to the standard treatments alone (averaged 48 hours to stop). By the end of four weeks, 100 percent of those given *S. boulardii* were cured of the amoeba, while 19 percent of those given the standard treatments continued to shed the amoeba in their stools.[50]

Conclusions and Observations for Acute Adult Diarrhea

Two probiotics have been shown to have some effectiveness for acute adult diarrhea. Adult diarrhea is a neglected area of research, but these studies focus attention on the possibilities of probiotic therapy.

Use of probiotics in adults was well tolerated and no serious adverse effects were noted. Further research is needed, and more probiotic strains should be tested for effectiveness.

Recommendations for Acute Adult Diarrhea

- Probiotic use may be worthwhile for adults with diarrhea of unknown cause.
- *S. boulardii* and *Enterococcus faecium* SF68 have the best evidence to support use.

Take the probiotic at the first sign of significant diarrhea and continue until the symptoms disappear.

OVERALL CONCLUSIONS

Most studies (see Figure 3.2) have shown probiotics to be effective in preventing acute pediatric diarrhea and treating acute adult diarrhea, but over one-third of all trials for the treatment of pediatric diarrhea did not show that probiotics were effective.

Want to get more technical information? Meta-analysis is a technique to evaluate a series of similar studies and give an overall estimate

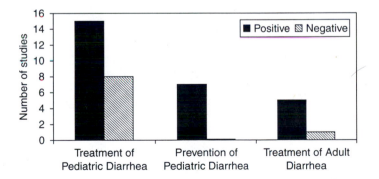

FIGURE 3.2. Comparison of the number of positive and negative randomized controlled trials showing clinical effectiveness for probiotics for acute diarrhea. Positive = effectiveness shown in controlled clinical trial, Negative = no significant effectiveness shown in controlled clinical trial.

of how effective a treatment is for all patients. Four meta-analyses found that probiotics could prevent an average of 40 percent of pediatric cases of diarrhea,[1,51-53] and one found that probiotics could prevent 34 percent of acute adult diarrhea.[54]

Chapter 4

Antibiotics-Associated Diarrhea and Colitis

One common adverse effect of antibiotics use is diarrhea. The medication itself may cause diarrhea or increase the susceptibility to infection by diarrhea-causing microbes. Since most of us take antibiotics at one time or another, knowledge of this adverse effect is helpful.

ANTIBIOTICS-ASSOCIATED DIARRHEA

Antibiotics are the most effective weapons available in the battle against infectious diseases, but their use is not without complications. One of the most common of these arises when antibiotics disrupt normal intestinal microflora, resulting in antibiotics-associated diarrhea (AAD). One of every five people who takes antibiotics develops this type of diarrhea. AAD is increasing in a wide variety of patient populations and is a serious concern for hospitalized patients. The microbial cause of AAD is known for only about one-third of the cases, so the use of drugs targeted to specific pathogens is of limited value. Probiotics offer a way to help reestablish the normal microbial flora disrupted by antibiotics and restore health.

Frequently Asked Questions

Is AAD serious?

It can be. Usually the episode does not last long, but more serious complications can develop. Up to 20 percent of those who develop AAD experience such complications.

Do some antibiotics cause AAD more frequently than others?

Yes. Antibiotics that are considered "broad-spectrum," that is, they target many different types of microbes, are associated with the greatest frequency of AAD. Also, antibiotics that target the anaerobic bacteria found in the lower bowel make the body more susceptible to AAD.

Why not just use low-risk antibiotics?

Low-risk, or "narrow-spectrum," antibiotics that target only a few types of infectious organisms are not always the most appropriate. Often, the cause of the infection cannot be quickly or easily identified, so a broad-spectrum antibiotic is needed. Frequently, several pathogens are involved in the infection process, so a broad-spectrum antibiotic is needed to inhibit as many types as possible. Even narrow-spectrum antibiotics (clindamycin and penicillin VK) can cause diarrhea.

When is the onset of AAD?

Diarrhea is a common side effect of antibiotics and usually begins within 24 to 48 hours of starting the antibiotic, but can be delayed for up to three months after stopping the antibiotics.

Do probiotics help prevent AAD?

Yes, they are one of the most effective methods to prevent AAD.

Epidemiology of AAD

Diarrhea is the most common adverse effect of antibiotic therapy. Several factors that increase the likelihood of acquiring AAD are shown in the following table. The reported frequency of AAD is as high as 26 percent (see Table 4.1), depending on the type of antibiotic, host factors (age, health status, and gender), hospitalization status, and presence of a nosocomial (hospital-acquired) outbreak.[17] Non-hospitalized, ambulatory (not confined to bed) patients usually experience the lowest frequency of AAD. A study of nonhospitalized adult members of a health maintenance organization found just 8

TABLE 4.1. Frequency of AAD in various populations.

Patient population	Country	Number in the study	Frequency*	Reference
Hospitalized patients				
Hospitalized patients	United States	136	29	Note 1
Adults in community hospital	United States	64	22	Note 2
Adults with respiratory or intestinal infections	France	388	18	Note 3
Community hospital patients	United States	96	15	Note 4
Adults	France	261	15.3	Note 5
Adults on infectious disease ward	France	240	13.3	Note 6
Patients given β-lactams	Thailand	140	10.7	Note 7
Patients given clindamycin	Thailand	140	8.6	Note 7
Adult surgery patients with prophylactic antibiotics	United Kingdom	180	8.4	Note 8
Children aged than five years	India	111	3.6	Note 9
Adults in tertiary care hospital	United States	NA	2.2	Note 10
Adults in tertiary care hospital	United States	NA	2.2	Note 11
Adults on OB/GYN service	United States	74,120	0.02	Note 12
Hospital Outbreaks				
Outbreak: general medicine	United States	399	25.8	Note 13
Outbreak: adult patients	Spain	386	5.9	Note 14
Outpatient populations				
Adults in HMO	United States	358,389	0.012	Note 15
Adults in HMO	United States	662,500	0.008	Note 16

*Frequency is per 100 people.

Abbreviations = AAD, antibiotic associated diarrhea; NA = data not available; HMO = health maintenance organization; OB/GYN = obstetrics and gynecology.

cases of AAD in 100,000 people per year.[16] Another study looked at 358,389 enrollees in four UnitedHealth Group plans over two years and found only 12 cases of AAD in 100,000 people annually.[15] These lower rates probably are due to the generally better health of outpatients compared to hospitalized patients, lack of exposure to pathogens that commonly contaminate hospital environments, and the use of milder antibiotics that do not kill off the protective microflora. Also, AAD may not have been reported unless it was very serious. The good news is the risk of AAD is relatively low for nonhospitalized adults. The bad news is the risk increases substantially for children and for those with the listed AAD risk factors, as shown in Table 4.2.

The highest rates of AAD are found in patients who are hospitalized. The normal frequency of AAD in hospitals may be as high as 29 percent. A study of 429 hospitalized patients receiving cefoperazone plus piperacillin found 29 percent developed AAD.[1] In 96 patients receiving β-lactam antibiotics at a community hospital, 14 (14.6 percent) developed AAD.[4]

AAD most frequently occurs during nosocomial (hospital-acquired) outbreaks when cases are clustered in time, exposure, susceptibility and proximity. Hospital outbreaks of AAD are to be expected when an inciting agent (antibiotics), an infectious agent and a susceptible patient population are intermixed. Most hospital outbreaks of AAD are due to *Clostridium difficile,* but AAD can stem from other causes. Outbreaks of hospital diarrhea also may be due to rotaviral infections, calicivirus and *Entamoeba histolytica,* but here the association with antibiotics is unclear. *C. difficile* is the only cause of AAD for which readily available diagnostic tools (strain identification, typing

TABLE 4.2. Factors that increase the risk of developing AAD.

Host factors	Environment	Medications	Medical procedures
Increasing age	Hospitalization	Broad-spectrum antibiotics	Surgery
Multiple types of infections	Long hospital stays	Multiple antibiotics	Enemas
Prior episodes of AAD	Roommates with diarrhea	Chemotherapy	Nasogastric tube feedings
Newborn baby			

techniques, culture assays, and environmental sampling techniques) are routinely used.[17]

Causes of AAD

AAD results from the disruption of normal intestinal flora by the antibiotic. This may result in two outcomes: Overgrowth by opportunistic pathogens and alterations of the flora's metabolic functions. "Colonization resistance," or the ability of normal flora to resist overgrowth by pathogenic organisms, has been well documented.[18] Colonization resistance operates on several levels within the intestinal tract:

- Competition for microbial nutrients
- Production of bacteriocins (microbial killing factors)
- Toxin-degrading proteases (enzymes that destroy disease-causing toxins)
- Blocking the infectious agent's attachment or toxin receptor sites

Colonization resistance results from the interactions of numerous microorganisms comprising a healthy, balanced microbial flora. Broad-spectrum antibiotics have the greatest destructive impact on intestinal flora. The risk for a specific antibiotic to cause AAD depends on two main factors: The spectrum of activity against normal flora and the degree of absorption from the intestinal tract. Narrow-spectrum antibiotics are associated with low rates of AAD because they do not disrupt many of the resident bacteria within the intestine and usually target only the pathogenic microbe. Broad-spectrum antibiotics, especially those affecting anaerobic flora (those bacteria that cannot tolerate oxygen), are associated with higher rates of AAD because they destroy not only the pathogenic microbe but many of the protective microbes normally found in the gut (see Figure 4.1). The degree of absorption also affects the frequency of AAD. Antibiotics (such as clindamycin) that are poorly absorbed from the colon or released in bile to reenter the intestine are associated with high rates of AAD because they have prolonged exposure to the microflora. Even antibiotics that are given intravenously (for example, cefoperazone and ampicillin) can cause AAD because they may be excreted in the bile

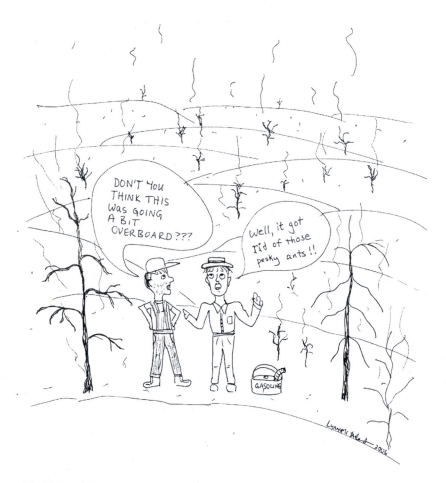

FIGURE 4.1. The "shot gun" effects of broad-spectrum antibiotics can be like a forest fire raging through the microbial flora of the intestines, clearing everything in its path. *Source:* Illustration by Lynne V. McFarland.

and may diffuse into the intestine from the bloodstream. Antibiotics with high absorption and little activity against the protective anaerobic microflora (for example, ciprofloxacin) produce lower rates of AAD. Once colonization resistance has been disrupted, overgrowth by opportunistic pathogens may occur. A number of important pathogens are capable of this opportunistic overgrowth. Some of these are listed in Table 4.3.

TABLE 4.3. Known causes of AAD.

Bacterial	Fungal	Metabolic alterations
Clostridium difficile	*Candida albicans*	Short-chain fatty acids
Klebsiella oxytoca		
Staphylococcus aureus		
Clostridium perfringens		

Clinical Features of AAD

The severity of AAD varies from uncomplicated diarrhea to colitis to pseudomembranous colitis (PMC).[19] Uncomplicated diarrhea is the most frequent result of AAD (10-30 per 100 patients), while colitis (which is more severe) is less frequent (5-10 per 100 patients) and PMC (the most severe form) is infrequent (<0.1 per 100 patients) but very serious. Diarrhea can be defined several ways, but an acceptable definition is a change in normal stool frequency with at least three loose or watery bowel movements for two days.[17,18] Symptoms may include low-grade fever, foul-smelling or greenish stools with or without mucus, and, rarely, the presence of blood in stools. The incubation period of AAD (the time between starting the antibiotic and the onset of diarrhea) falls into two groups: Early onset, occurring during antibiotic use, and delayed onset, which may occur from two to eight weeks after antibiotics have been discontinued. In a study of patients on β-lactam antibiotics (such as penicillins and cephalosporins), the average incubation period for AAD was 14 days but ranged from 2 to 55 days.[4] Most patients developed AAD while on the antibiotics (62 percent); however, more than one-third did not develop AAD until after the antibiotics had been discontinued. The average duration of AAD was four days if diarrhea occurred while the person was taking antibiotics, and 18 days if AAD occurred post antibiotics.

Consequences of AAD

Consequences of AAD include extended hospital stays, increases in rates of subsequent infections, and higher medical costs.[20] Development of AAD in hospital patients increases the risk of developing another type of infection (usually of the urinary tract) fivefold.[21] AAD can be sufficiently severe to necessitate hospitalization even for ambulatory patients who are normally at low risk. In one study of hospitalized patients, the average stay was significantly longer (35 days) for patients with diarrhea compared to patients without diarrhea (19 days, $p = 0.01$).[20] The investigators reported a trend for higher mortality rates in patients with AAD compared to controls, but no specific cause of death was more common than others.

Treatments for AAD

Discontinuation of Inciting Antibiotics

For uncomplicated cases of AAD, the most prudent measure is to discontinue or change the inciting antibiotic, if possible. People often take antibiotics when they are not needed, as in the case of antibiotics for the flu. Any disease caused by a virus, such as a cold or influenza, is not affected by antibiotics. If significant diarrhea develops while taking an antibiotic and signs of the infection are gone, it may be best to stop the antibiotic. However, it is important to consult your medical provider before doing so because some infections need to be treated vigorously to avoid a rebound of disease and to limit the development of antibiotic resistance. For serious cases of AAD, active treatment is required.

Antibiotic Treatment

In instances where the cause of AAD is known, specific antibiotics targeted against these pathogens are recommended. For example, if *Candida* is found, treatment with oral nystatin or fluconazole should clear this pathogen within a week. Usually, however, the causative pathogen is unknown.

Prevention of AAD by Probiotics

AAD is a direct effect of antibiotic killing of normal bacteria, so prevention of AAD has traditionally focused on limiting the overuse and abuse of antibiotics. Antibiotics are overprescribed for viral respiratory infections and bronchitis, and overuse is associated with an increase in antibiotic resistance. Probiotics offer a different modality to prevent AAD, an approach that may allow the course of antibiotic therapy to be completed and the infection cured without the patient experiencing diarrhea. This approach is routinely used in Europe for patients who are given antibiotics. The use of probiotics to prevent AAD has been highly successful, as shown by the studies in Table 4.4. Several review articles have concluded that probiotics have been efficacious for the prevention of AAD.[22-24] For example, a review of seven placebo-controlled, randomized studies found that probiotics reduce the risk of AAD by more than a third.[25] Two advantages of using probiotics with antibiotics are: The use of probiotics minimizes the impact of the antibiotic on the normal intestinal flora, and probiotics have a low risk of adverse effects (covered in Chapter 8).

Saccharomyces boulardii. The strongest evidence for the role of living organisms in the treatment of AAD comes from randomized controlled clinical trials involving the probiotic yeast *S. boulardii*. This has been studied in five large blinded trials for the prevention of AAD (see Table 4.4) and found to be significantly effective in four of the five and very well tolerated.[2-4,31] One study at a Seattle, WA, hospital enrolled patients who were starting a new prescription of antibiotics.[2] The patients were randomized to receive capsules containing the yeast or a placebo along with the antibiotic. The study treatment began within 48 hours of the start of the antibiotic and continued two weeks after the last antibiotic dose to give time for the normal intestinal microflora to recover from the antibiotic. Of the 180 enrolled patients, significantly fewer (9.5 percent) on the probiotic developed AAD compared to those receiving placebo (21.8 percent). The probiotic was well tolerated by the patients.

In another study, 193 hospitalized patients receiving at least one β-lactam antibiotic (such as penicillins or cephalosporins) were treated with *S. boulardii* or placebo for four weeks. Fewer cases of AAD were observed in the *S. boulardii* group (7.2 percent) compared to the placebo group (14.6 percent), and no serious adverse effects were observed.[4] A third trial was conducted in France with 388 patients randomized to a fairly low dose of *S. boulardii* (200 mg/day) or placebo along with their antibiotic for seven days.[3] Again, fewer patients given *S. boulardii* developed AAD (4.5 percent) compared to patients given placebo (17.5 percent). A study in children who were taking

TABLE 4.4. Probiotics for the prevention of Antibiotics-Associated Diarrhea.

Probiotic	Population	Daily dose	Duration (days)	AAD in the probiotic group	AAD in the controls	Reference
Clostridium butyricum MIYAIRI	110 children on mostly cephalosporins or penicillin	ng	6	7%*	59%	Note 26
Lactobacillus GG	81 hospitalized children	1×10^{10}	Varied	6.7%*	33.3%	Note 27
Lactobacillus GG	267 hospitalized adults	2×10^{10}	14	29.3% ns	29.9%	Note 28
Lactobacillus GG	119 children on one antibiotic	4×10^{10}	14	5%*	16%	Note 29
Lactobacillus GG	188 outpatient children	2×10^{10}	10	7%*	26%	Note 30
S. boulardii	69 elderly patients	4.5×10^{9}	14	21% ns	13.9%	Note 31
S. boulardii	193 hospitalized adults (one or more beta-lactam antibiotics)	2×10^{10}	28	7.2%*	14.6%	Note 4
S. boulardii	180 hospitalized adults	2×10^{10}	28	9.5%*	21.8%	Note 2
S. boulardii	388 hospitalized adults	4×10^{9}	7	4.5%*	17.5%	Note 3
S. boulardii	246 children	1×10^{10}	Varied	3.4%*	17.3%	Note 32
L. Acidophilus & L. bulgaricus	38 children on amoxicillin	4 g	10	66% ns	69.5%	Note 33
L. Acidophilus & L. bulgaricus	79 hospitalized adults, mostly on ampicillin	4 g	5	0%*	14%	Note 34
Enterococcus faecium SF68	45 adult patients	1.5×10^{7}	7	8.7% ns	27.2%	Note 35

*$p < 0.05$.

Abbreviations: ns = not significant; ng = data not given; g = grams.

antibiotics for ear or respiratory infections was designed so that half received *S. boulardii* (500 mg/day) and the other half received placebo.[32] The frequency of diarrhea in the probiotic group was only 3.4 percent compared to 17.3 percent in the placebo group. The yeast probiotic was well tolerated by the children. A smaller study using a lower dose of the yeast for elderly patients taking antibiotics did not show benefit of the yeast in reducing AAD.[31]

A significant advantage of this yeast probiotic is it is not inhibited by antibiotics and can be given simultaneously with them. Antibiotics inhibit only bacteria, not yeasts. In contrast, other bacterial probiotics must be chosen and dosed with care, as the antibiotic being used by the patient may also affect or kill the living bacterial probiotics. Bacterial probiotics should be taken at least two hours before or after the antibiotic to help maintain probiotic activity.

Lactobacilli probiotics. Several *Lactobacillus* strains have been tested for the prevention of AAD. A commercial mixture of *Lactobacillus acidophilus* and *L. bulgaricus* (Lactinex) was not successful in preventing AAD in two studies.[33,34] Of the four studies testing *Lactobacillus rhamnosus* GG, three showed this strain of probiotic was effective in preventing AAD. A study of 119 children in Finland who were receiving just one type of antibiotic were given *Lactobacillus rhamnosus* GG or placebo for two weeks.[29] Fewer children treated with *Lactobacillus* GG (5 percent) developed AAD compared to the children receiving placebo (16 percent). Two other studies of children also showed significant protection by this probiotic.[30,36] Interestingly, when *Lactobacillus* GG was tried in 267 hospitalized adult patients receiving antibiotics, no difference in AAD rates between those getting the probiotic or placebo was noted.[28] The adult patients in this study received the probiotic for a similar duration and at a similar dose as the children, so researchers speculated that the hospitalized adult patients may have received different types of antibiotics (for example, powerful intravenous antibiotics) from the pediatric patients, who received drugs but were not hospitalized.

Other probiotics. Two other probiotic strains have been tested for prevention of AAD: *Clostridium butyricum* subspecies MIYAIRI and *Enterococcus faecium* SF68. One study randomized 110 children, who were mostly on cephalosporins or penicillins, to six days of *Clostridium butyricum* subspecies MIYAIRI or placebo.[26] Significantly fewer (7 percent) children on the clostridial probiotic developed AAD compared to the children given placebo (59 percent). *Enterococcus faecium* SF68 was tested in 45 adult patients at a low dose (10^7 organisms/day), and this reduced frequency of AAD in those given the probiotic to 9 percent, compared to 27 percent of those given placebo.[35]

Recommendations for Prevention of AAD

- An appropriate probiotic should be routinely used with an antibiotic to prevent AAD.
- Probiotic use should begin as soon as possible after starting antibiotic therapy and continued for one week after the antibiotic is stopped.
- Probiotics with the best evidence for prevention of AAD are *Lactobacillus rhamnosus* GG and *Saccharomyces boulardii.*

CLOSTRIDIUM DIFFICILE *AAD*

A specific type of AAD is *Clostridium difficile* AAD (abbreviated CD-AAD). This usually is discussed as a separate illness because its mechanism and the treatments are specific to this disease. Unlike most types of AAD, where the microbe causing the illness is not known, the bacterium that causes this type of AAD has been well researched and tests are available for its detection.

Frequently Asked Questions about Clostridium difficile AAD

What is the difference between AAD and Clostridium difficile *AAD?*

AAD caused by *Clostridium difficile* may be more severe than other forms of AAD.

Where is Clostridium difficile *AAD found?*

It is found mostly in hospitalized patients.

What types of infections can Clostridium difficile *cause?*

People may be colonized by the *C. difficile* bacteria and have no symptoms (asymptomatic carriers) or may have mild diarrhea. In more severe cases, inflammatory diarrhea is found with fever and can develop into colitis. *C. difficile* colitis can be lethal in rare cases.

How long does Clostridium difficile *AAD last?*

Usually, the diarrhea lasts one to two weeks with treatment, but it may develop into a recurrent form of the disease, which may persist for years.

Is Clostridium difficile *found in other species?*

Yes, *Clostridium difficile* disease has occurred in horses, bears, dogs, cats, and several other mammals.

Are probiotics effective for Clostridium difficile *AAD?*

So far, only one probiotic, *Saccharomyces boulardii,* has been shown to be effective.

Epidemiology of Clostridium difficile *AAD*

Clostridium difficile is one of the leading causes of diarrhea outbreaks in hospitals. The microbe is a gram-positive bacterial rod that produces spores (see Figure 4.2) resistant to disinfectants commonly used in hospitals. Numerous outbreaks of *C. difficile*-associated AAD (CD-AAD) have been reported internationally since the 1980s, with the number of cases ranging from 15 to 78 patients during outbreaks.

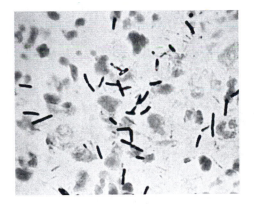

FIGURE 4.2. Microbiologic appearance of *Clostridium difficile* (dark purple rods) in a stool sample with inflammatory debris and white blood cells (stained red). Spores of *Clostridium difficile* can be seen as clear circles within the dark bacterial rods. *Source:* Photo by Lynne V. McFarland.

Early studies of CD-AAD hospital outbreaks successfully documented that this organism can be transmitted by roommates and hospital personnel, and indirectly contaminate environmental sources, resulting in new infections.[17] Mothers of newborns sometimes develop a recurrent form of CD-AAD due to repeated exposures to contaminated diapers.[37] Newborns pick up *C. difficile* quite easily while they are at the hospital, but usually do not develop symptoms and appear healthy. If the mother has received antibiotics in the hospital, her intestinal microbes are disrupted and she is at greater risk of contracting *C. difficile* from her baby.

In 2004, over 100 people died of CD-AAD in Ontario, Canada

CD-AAD came to the attention of the medical community when the frequency of hospital outbreaks began to increase. Up to half of all hospital AAD cases and nearly all (95 to 99 percent) cases of PMC can be attributed to *C. difficile*.[20] Overgrowth by *C. difficile* results in disease due to the action of three toxins called toxin A, toxin B, and binary toxin. These toxins cause the normally rectangular cells that line the intestinal tract (enterocytes) to lose their shape. The change in shape of the intestinal lining cells causes gaps to form in the inner layer of the intestinal wall, which leads to fluid leakage and diarrhea. In addition to the physical disruption of enterocytes, toxins A and B attract polymorphonuclear leukocytes (white blood cells) and other inflammatory cells to the site, which is why this type of diarrhea is considered inflammatory. Although *C. difficile* causes up to 50 percent of hospital AAD cases, other possible causes exist but they are not as well studied.

Clinical Features of CD-AAD

The spectrum of CD-AAD diseases ranges from asymptomatic carriage (no diarrhea) to uncomplicated diarrhea (no inflammation or fever) to colitis (inflammation and fever) to the most severe form, PMC, which can be life-threatening. Other abdominal symptoms (cramping or discomfort) may accompany diarrhea. If colitis develops, diarrhea usually is more severe and accompanied by abdominal pain or cramping, fever that exceeds 104°F, hypoalbuminemia (low protein in the blood), and leukocytosis (increase in white blood cells).[38] Colitis has to be diagnosed by a physician using a colonoscope that allows for both the examination of the internal surface of the intestine and for a biopsy to be taken. Colitis is diagnosed if the biopsy shows inflammatory changes (redness, swelling, or damage of the cells) and no pseudomembranes are seen on the intestinal wall. It also is diagnosed if microscopic examination finds "summit lesions" or "volcano lesions" (inflammatory cells and debris ejected into the colonic lumen). At the extreme end of the severity spectrum is pseudomembranous colitis (PMC), which almost always is associated with *C. difficile*. Common symptoms of PMC include watery diarrhea (90-95 percent), abdominal cramping (80-90 percent), fever (80 percent), increase in white blood cells (80 percent), and, rarely, vomiting. Most patients with PMC develop symptoms within a week of antibiotic exposure, but onset of symptoms in as many as 40 percent of patients may be delayed two to eight weeks after antibiotics have been discontinued. PMC is diagnosed when an endoscopic examination reveals white to yellow plaques or a layer of a pseudomembrane in the colon (see Figure 4.3). Complications of PMC may

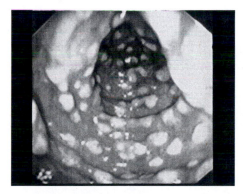

Pseudomembranous Colitis

FIGURE 4.3. Endoscopic examination of the colon in cases of pseudomembranous colitis reveals yellow-white plaques and swelling of the intestinal tissue. *Source:* Photograph provided courtesy of Christina Surawicz, MD, Harborview Medical Center, Seattle, WA.

include hypocalcemia (low calcium, 37 percent), kidney failure (27 percent), and hypoproteinema (low protein levels, 50 percent). Less frequently, PMC complications may include toxic megacolon, Reiter's syndrome, perforation of the colon, shock, or death. In some cases, surgery is required to remove the colon.

Recurrent CD-AAD

Usually patients have just one episode of *Clostridium difficile,* which is successfully treated with antibiotics. However, one in five patients goes on to develop chronic, recurrent CD-AAD. This form of CD-AAD has been noted in 20 percent of patients after their initial episode has been treated, and recurrent episodes may persist for up to four years despite multiple treatments with antibiotics.[39,40] Once a person has at least two episodes of CD-AAD, the probability of more episodes increases dramatically to 65 percent. There is no reliable method to predict who will develop this form of recurrent disease, so it is important to try and find an effective treatment quickly. Since standard antibiotics alone do not cure recurrent CD-AAD, probiotics have a useful role as an adjunctive (or add-on) therapy.

Consequences *of* Clostridium difficile *Infections*

The consequences of CD-AAD infections are well documented. Hospitalized patients with CD-AAD had an average extended stay of one to three weeks. Because these patients usually are treated with high-dose vancomycin, CD-AAD infections have been associated with more vancomycin-resistant enterococcal infections in hospitals.[41] The recurrent form of CD-AAD leads to increased use and cost of antibiotics, especially vancomycin, additional hospitalizations, and other medical complications.[40] Less frequent but catastrophic complications include multiple organ failure, reactive arthritis, and sepsis (spread to the blood) with *C. difficile.* According to one study, medical costs (bed, laboratory tests, and treatments) averaged $2,000 to $5,000 per patient for each episode of CD-AAD.[42] Mortality from 3.5 to 10 percent has been reported for hospitalized patients with CD-AAD, compared with mortality rates of 4 to 7 percent for other hospitalized patients without CD-AAD. Mortality increases to 30 to 43 percent in surgical patients with *C. difficile* colitis or PMC. These mortality rates may reflect the diminished health of hospitalized patients who undergo invasive surgery or are severely ill, and may be merely a surrogate measure of more severely ill patients rather than a true increased risk of mortality for patients with CD-AAD.

Treatments for Clostridium difficile AAD

Discontinuation of Inciting Antibiotic

For uncomplicated cases of *Clostridium difficile,* the most prudent measure is to discontinue or change the inciting antibiotic, if possible. Often, people take antibiotics when they are not needed. Antibiotics have no effect on viral disease, such as colds or flu. If there is no justified reason to take an antibiotic, discontinue it. Sometimes the antibiotic can be discontinued because the symptoms are mild, and diarrhea may pose a greater risk. In a review of CD-AAD cases over ten years, this approach was effective in 15 percent of the 908 cases.[43] However, for more serious cases of AAD and CD-AAD, more active treatment is required.

Antibiotic Treatment for CD-AAD

Vancomycin and metronidazole are recommended for the standard treatment of *C. difficile.*[44] In a randomized study of 119 patients with CD-AAD testing four antibiotics, clinical cures were similar for vancomycin (94 percent), metronidazole (94 percent), teicoplanin (96 percent), and fusidic acid (93 percent).[45] The latter two antibiotics are not routinely used in the United States. Studies continue to show similar effectiveness for vancomycin and metronidazole.[46] Vancomycin has been shown to be more effective in reducing the duration of diarrhea (by an average of three days) compared to metronidazole (by an average of five days). Currently, however, oral vancomycin is not recommended as a first line of treatment for patients with initial CD-AAD or AAD infections because it is expensive and routine use may lead to resistance to this powerful, life-saving drug.[46] Vancomycin use should be restricted to patients who have previously failed on metronidazole, carry a metronidazole-resistant strain, are allergic to metronidazole, pregnant, or severely ill with PMC or toxic megacolon.

A more difficult treatment problem is recurrent CD-AAD. In one study, recurrence rates of 28 percent with fusidic acid, 16 percent with vancomycin or metronidazole, and 7 percent with teicoplanin were reported.[45] In 34 patients with a history of CD-AAD, the recurrence rate within two months of antibiotic treatment with either vancomycin or metronidazole was 64.7 percent.[46] Strategies of antibiotic treatment for recurrent CD-AAD include a repeat course of antibiotic using a prolonged, tapering dose schedule or a pulsed (every other day) scheme.[47,48] Surgery may be a treatment of last resort for some patients with severe cases of CD-AAD and incurable PMC. The desire for an effective treatment that would not further perturb the colon flora (as with an additional course of antibiotics) has generated interest in nonantibiotic treatments. What is needed is a treatment strategy that would help reestablish normal flora (and colonization resistance) while limiting the use of additional antibiotics. Probiotics offer this treatment strategy.

Probiotics for the Treatment of Clostridium difficile AAD

Several randomized controlled trials have shown that probiotics can be very effective in the treatment of CD-AAD (see Table 4.5). Probiotics for this disease are used to treat patients who are already ill with diarrhea and have been diagnosed with *Clostridium difficile*. Most studies have not relied solely on the probiotic to cure this serious form of AAD; rather, they have combined the probiotic with one of the antibiotics that are commonly used to treat CD-AAD (either vancomycin or metronidazole). This combination therapy has been tested because treatment of CD-AAD with standard antibiotics alone has not been effective in 20 percent of the cases.

Since CD-AAD is due to an overgrowth of *C. difficile* because of antibiotic disruption of the protective normal intestinal microflora, the goal of therapy should be to both kill the *C. difficile* and help restore the normal flora (see Figure 4.4). Probiotics combined with effective antibiotics against *C. difficile* can fulfill this goal as well as restore normal protective colonic microflora. Furthermore, some probiotics produce substances that act directly against the pathogenic organisms or their toxins. Thus, probiotics can be an effective partner with antibiotic therapy for CD-AAD.

Saccharomyces boulardii. Early studies with *S. boulardii* showed the first promising results for the use of probiotics in CD-AAD (Table 4.3). Two studies that gave *S. boulardii* to small numbers of children or adults were encouraging, but these were not placebo-controlled

TABLE 4.5. Probiotics in the treatment of *Clostridium difficile* Antibiotics-Associated Diarrhea.

Probiotic	Population	Daily dose	Duration (days)	Frequency of CD-AAD relapses in the probiotic group	Frequency of CD-AAD relapses in the controls	Reference
Controlled trials						
S. boulardii	32 adult patients on vancomycin (2 g/d)	2×10^{10}	28	17%*	50%	Note 47
S. boulardii	124 adult patients on varied doses of vancomycin or metronidazole	2×10^{10}	28	26.3%*	44.8%	Note 46
Lactobacillus rhamnosus GG	25 adults on vancomycin or metronidazole	ng	21	36.4% ns	35.7%	Note 49
L. plantarum 299v	20 adults	5×10^{10}	38	36% ns	67%	Note 50
Case series						
S. boulardii	13 adults	2×10^{10}	30	15%	No controls	Note 51
S. boulardii	19 infants	Varied	15	95%	No controls	Note 52
Lactobacillus rhamnosus GG	5 adults with recurrent CD-AAD	1×10^{10}	7–10	20%	No controls	Note 53
Lactobacillus rhamnosus GG	4 infants	1.2×10^{9}	14	50%	No controls	Note 54
Lactobacillus rhamnosus GG	32 adults patients	2×10^{9}	21	15.6%	No controls	Note 55
S. cerevisiae	3 adults	ng	14	0%	No controls	Note 56

*$p < 0.05$.

Abbreviations: ns = not significant; ng = data not given; g = grams; mg = milligrams; d = day.

trials, so further research was needed before a firm conclusion could be reached.[52,57] Additional studies were launched to see if this benefit could be demonstrated more convincingly in controlled clinical trials. The first randomized, placebo-controlled trial involved 124 patients with CD-AAD and tested the addition of *S. boulardii* to standard anti-

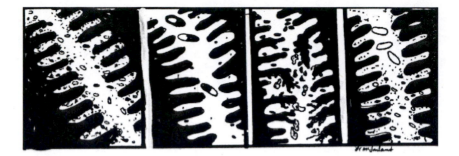

FIGURE 4.4. Restoration of normal protective microbial flora with probiotic treatment is shown. Panels from the left to right: (1) a healthy intestine showing a rich diversity of microbes acting as a barrier to infection by pathogenic bacteria, (2) an antibiotic-treated intestine showing elimination of much of the protective flora, (3) an antibiotic-treated intestine showing an invasion of opportunistic pathogenic bacteria, such as *clostridium difficile*, and (4) an intestine treated with probiotics to restore the protective microbial flora. *Source:* Illustration by Lynne V. McFarland.

biotic treatment.[46] In the group treated with *S. boulardii,* further recurrences of CD-AAD were significantly reduced (26 percent) when compared to a placebo-standard antibiotic group (45 percent). This finding was confirmed in a later study of adults who had recurrent *Clostridium difficile* disease and were treated over ten days with either a high dose of vancomycin (2g/day), a low dose of vancomycin (500 mg/day), or metronidazole (1 g/day).[47] Patients were randomized to *S. boulardii* or placebo for four weeks, and then were followed an additional four weeks to see if they had further recurrences of CD-AAD. Only the combination of high-dose vancomycin and *S. boulardii* was effective for this group of patients. Neither the lower dose of vancomycin nor metronidazole eliminated *Clostridium difficile* toxins at the end of the ten-day treatment, and this may be why these groups did not improve. These studies show that, for serious recurrent CD-AAD, a very vigorous antibiotic treatment together with the probiotic is needed.

Lactobacillus strains. Lactobacillus rhamnosus GG was reported to reduce recurrences of CD-AAD in a study of four children.[54] Another researcher used *Lactobacillus* GG in milk to successfully treat five adult patients with recurrent CD-AAD.[53] However, both studies tested only small numbers of patients and there were no control groups. At the time of writing this book, there was only one placebo-controlled trial using *Lactobacillus* GG for treating recurrent CD-AAD.[49] In this study, 25 adults with recurrent CD-AAD were treated with either vancomycin or metronidazole, and randomized to *Lactobacillus* GG or placebo for three weeks. The recurrence rate was the same for the probiotic group (36 percent) and the placebo (36 percent). The authors did not report the doses of the standard antibiotic used, so perhaps the reason this trial did not show effectiveness is similar to that of the previously discussed study,[47] where no effect was observed with metronidazole or the low-dose vancomycin. Further studies are needed to establish the effectiveness of *Lactobacillus* GG for CD-AAD. Another small randomized trial was conducted treating 20 adults with either *L. plantarum* 299v or placebo for 38 days.[50] There was no significant difference in the two groups.

Other combination treatments with probiotics. Another yeast (*Saccharomyces cerevisiae,* or baker's yeast) was tested in a small case series (Table 4.5), but as this study did not have a control group, no firm conclusions can be drawn. Another tactic has been investigated for patients with recurrent CD-AAD who may have low levels of protective antibodies against *Clostridium difficile.* A researcher gave one such patient pooled immunoglobulin as treatment.[58] This patient with recurrent CD-AAD was successfully treated when intravenous immune globulin had been added to her therapy with vancomycin and *S. boulardii.* This area of combined probiotic, antibiotic, and immunoglobulin therapy is an interesting approach but needs further research to define its potential.

Recommendations for CD-AAD

- Both antibiotics and probiotics should be used for CD-AAD. The antibiotics kill the *C. difficile,* and the probiotics help restore the protective intestinal flora.
- The probiotic should be started as soon as the diagnosis of CD-AAD is established and continued for four to six weeks after diarrhea has stopped.
- *Saccharomyces boulardii* has the best evidence to support its use for CD-AAD.

More Technical Reviews

A more technical method to combine many studies and get a combined estimate of how well a treatment does for a similar disease is called meta-analysis. Five meta-analyses show probiotics can prevent an average of 43 percent of AAD cases and 59 percent of CD-AAD cases.[24, 25,59-61]

CONCLUSIONS

Cases of AAD are becoming more frequent due to increased use of broad-spectrum antibiotics, the aging of the population, and the increasing frequency of hospital outbreaks. Four major factors increase the risk of AAD and CD-AAD: host characteristics (age and comorbidity), environmental sources (shared hospital rooms, prolonged hospital stays, and outbreaks), increased use of medications (antibiotics or chemotherapy), and procedures (surgery and enemas). AAD may result in increased costs of medical care and has infrequent but serious complications, especially when caused by *C. difficile*. Further research into treatments and preventive measures is required.

As shown in Figure 4.5, 9 of the 13 randomized controlled trials had a positive effect for the prevention of AAD with probiotic use. Of

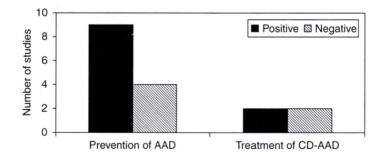

FIGURE 4.5. Comparison of the number of positive and negative randomized controlled trials showing clinical effectiveness for probiotics in various types of antibiotic associated diarrhea. Abbreviations: AAD = antibiotic-associated diarrhea, CD-AAD = *Clostridium difficile* antibiotic-associated diarrhea. Positive = effectiveness shown in controlled clinical trial, and Negative = no significant effectiveness shown in controlled clinical trial.

the four randomized controlled trials for CD-AAD, two probiotics (*S. boulardii* and *L. plantarum*) showed significant effectiveness. Probiotics offer an effective and safe method for both the prevention and treatment of AAD and the more serious recurrent CD-AAD.

Chapter 5

Vaginal and Urinary Tract Infections

With an estimated ten million office visits per year[1] in the United States, vaginitis is one of the most common reasons women see a gynecologist. A vaginal infection usually is first noticed as an abnormal discharge. Irritation, burning on urination, itching, and difficulty during sexual intercourse may be experienced. Urinary tract infections (UTI) generally affect women, although men with diminished urine flow or prostate hypertrophy may acquire a UTI. UTI are common, and although easily treated, are frustrating when they continue to recur. Probiotics are potentially helpful for some forms of vaginal infections and recurrent UTI.

BACTERIAL VAGINOSIS

In women of childbearing years, bacterial vaginosis (BV) and candida vaginitis are the most common vaginal infections. The vulva and cervix are less commonly involved. In contrast, sexually transmitted diseases such as gonorrhea and chlamydia involve the cervix, while herpes involves the vulva. An accurate diagnosis is important because the treatments for BV, candida vaginitis, and sexually transmitted diseases are vastly different. Only BV and candida vaginitis will be discussed in this chapter because probiotics have some application for these vaginal infections.

The Power of Probiotics
© 2007 by The Haworth Press, Inc. All rights reserved.
doi:10.1300/5597_05

Frequently Asked Questions

What is BV?

Bacterial vaginosis (BV) is a vaginal infection due to an overgrowth of certain pathogens and also due to a diminished number of protective lactobacilli.

What are the symptoms of BV?

Most women with BV have a "fishy" smelling vaginal discharge, but there may be no symptoms. An accurate diagnosis is needed so that effective treatments can be provided.

How is BV treated?

BV usually is treated with antibiotics.

If a woman is pregnant, can BV be harmful to the fetus?

Yes. BV can cause premature labor and other problems in pregnant women.

Are probiotics effective against BV?

Probiotics can help in the treatment and, especially, the prevention of BV.

BV is a common bacterial infection of the vagina. It is the most common cause of an abnormal vaginal discharge, accounting for about 40 percent of vaginitis cases.[1] It is a complex infection involving more than one pathogen. The primary pathogens involved are *Gardnerella vaginalis—mobiluncus* species and a variety of other gram-negative anaerobes. A discussion on the differences of gram-positive and gram-negative bacteria is found in Chapter 1.

A healthy vagina is populated by many strains of lactobacilli, especially those that produce hydrogen peroxide and lactic acid. The acid keeps the pH of the vaginal fluids low (acidic), and together with hydrogen peroxide production and the presence of lactobacilli, it maintains an environment that does not foster overgrowth of pathogens.

For reasons that are not completely understood, a change may take place that results in absent or diminished numbers of lactobacilli and an overgrowth of anaerobic gram-negative rods. The vaginal fluid pH increases, which facilitates overgrowth of these anaerobes, and the amines they generate give the secretions a fishy odor. This usually is the first complaint of a person with BV. Itching and irritation are commonly experienced as well, although many women have no overt symptoms at all. From a sample of vaginal fluid, a physician can diagnose BV by the elevated pH, fishy smell, and the presence of "clue cells" visible under a microscope. Clue cells are cells from the lining of the vagina that are surrounded or coated by gram-negative rods, as shown in Figure 5.1. A microscopic examination of a healthy vaginal fluid sample would show mostly gram-positive rods, a characteristic of lactobacilli.

While the symptoms of BV usually are mild, it can have severe consequences for the woman and, if she is pregnant, the unborn fetus. BV increases the risk of acquiring pelvic inflammatory disease as well as susceptibility to HIV infection and other sexually transmitted diseases.[2,3] BV during pregnancy increases the risk for premature labor, premature rupture of membranes, and preterm birth.[4-6] However, not all premature births can be attributed to infections, but BV and other infections do play a role in some premature births. Since BV can be present without obvious symptoms, the mother and physi-

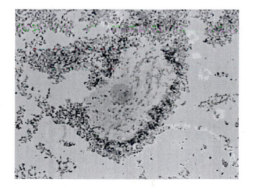

FIGURE 5.1. Microscopic slide of a clue cell, a diagnostic sign for bacterial vaginosis. *Source:* Davis D. Bacterial vaginosis guidance document. Available at http://www.fda.gov/cder/present/anti-infective798/bv/sld002.htm, 1998.

cian may not be aware of the infection and premature birth may occur with no apparent reason.

Antibiotic Treatments for BV

Treatment of BV with antibiotics is relatively straightforward. Metronidazole, which has strong activity against anaerobes, usually is successful, although it has adverse effects such as headache, a bad taste, and an increased risk for a vaginal yeast infection. Topical application of a cream containing antibiotics, such as clindamycin, targeted against anaerobic bacteria also can be used. Recurrence of BV after discontinuing antibiotics is common, with 50 percent of women having another infection within six months.[7] It is important to note that one study showed that antimicrobial treatment of pregnant women with asymptomatic BV did not decrease the risk of premature labor.[8] In developing countries, antimicrobials may not be readily available and untreated BV also plays a role in HIV acquisition. Therefore, there is a strong need for a therapeutic approach to prevent BV recurrences after antibiotic treatment and, most importantly, to prevent BV during pregnancy.

Probiotics and BV

The rationale for use of probiotics during pregnancy to prevent BV is compelling. BV is a culmination of imbalanced and "diseased" vaginal microflora characterized by low numbers of lactobacilli and high numbers of gram-negative anaerobic pathogens. If the high levels of lactic acid and hydrogen-peroxide-producing lactobacilli could be restored, BV recurrences would be infrequent because of the unfavorable environment for pathogen overgrowth. An inexpensive probiotic effective for BV could have benefits, on a global scale, by decreasing premature births, sexually transmitted disease risks, and HIV infections in developing countries. The ideal probiotic microbe would be inexpensive to produce, readily available for use in developing countries, taken orally, and promote high concentrations of lactic acid and hydrogen-peroxide-producing lactobacilli in the vaginal tract, which would produce pathogen-inhibitory substances. Although this ideal has not yet been achieved, studies evaluating the probiotic approach for BV control show considerable promise.

Early studies with no controls or comparison groups suggested that probiotics were useful for treating women with symptomatic BV. Researchers reported certain favorable effects by intravaginal administration of a live-culture yogurt to 34 women with BV,[9] but a placebo yogurt was not used in this study. Controlled studies for probiotic treatment of BV have been published (see Table 5.1). A well-designed study in Sweden used a H_2O_2 (hydrogen peroxide)-producing strain of *Lactobacillus acidophilus* in a suppository form to treat 57 women with BV.[10] At the end of the six-day treatment, 16 of the 28 probiotics-treated women (57 percent) had normal microbiologic results. This did not occur for any of the women treated with placebo. Most patients had a recurrence of BV after the next menstruation, which might indicate a need for longer treatments. Other studies tested in 32 patients with BV the efficacy of a vaginal tablet containing a hydrogen peroxide strain of *Lactobacillus acidophilus* and 0.03 mg estriol (Gynoflor).[11] Patients either received one to two probiotic tablets per day for six days or placebo tablets. Two weeks after the start of therapy, the cure rate in the probiotics-treated group was 77 percent, compared to just 25 percent ($p < 0.05$) in the placebo group. However, a control tablet containing only estriol was not tested, so the role of the probiotic *Lactobacillus* in the cure is not definitive.

TABLE 5.1. Probiotics for bacterial vaginosis (BV).

Probiotic	Number of patients in the study	Dose form	Time of treatment	Result*	Reference
L. acidophilus (La)	57 with BV	Vaginal suppository	Six days	57% cured at six days on La, 0% cured on placebo	Note 10
L. acidophilus (La) plus estriol	32 with BV	Vaginal tablet	Six days	88% cured at four weeks on La, 22% on placebo	Note 11
L. acidophilus (La)	20 with recurrent BV	Oral yogurt	Two months	25% had BV at one month on La, 50% had BV on placebo	Note 12
L. rhamnosus GR-1 and *L. fermentum* RC-14	64 healthy women	Oral capsules	Two months	0% on probiotic, developed BV, 25% on placebo, developed BV	Note 13

*All four trials found that the probiotics-treated women had significantly less BV than controls.

Evidence shows that probiotics might help prevent BV. Investigators in Israel conducted a study for prevention of recurrent candidal vaginitis and recurrent BV,[12] which compared women ingesting yogurt enriched with a hydrogen-peroxide-producing strain of *Lactobacillus acidophilus* with women ingesting pasteurized yogurt (control group). At one month, 25 percent of the women in the lactobacilli-treated group had an episode of BV, compared to 50 percent of the women in the control group. The *Lactobacillus acidophilus* strain in the yogurt was present in the vaginal fluid of most of the women ingesting the active yogurt, which shows that an orally administered probiotic can migrate from the intestines (specifically, the anus) and ascend into the vaginal tract. This study also showed that a therapeutic effect in the vaginal tract can be achieved by a probiotic administered orally.

Researchers in Toronto, Canada, have studied the role of vaginal lactobacilli in protecting against BV and urinary tract infections (UTI). They recently worked with two strains—*L. rhamnosus* GR-1 and *L. fermentum* RE-14—that can colonize the vagina after being taken orally.[13,14] In a double-blind, placebo-controlled clinical study, capsules containing either freeze-dried *L. rhamnosus* GR-1 and *L. fermentum* RC-14 or placebo were given to healthy women with no outward symptoms of BV for at least two months. Microbiological evaluation of the vaginal swabs revealed that more women who were negative for BV at the start of the study had BV at day 35 if they were in the placebo group (6 out of 24, 25 percent) compared to none of the 23 in the probiotics-treated group. More women in the probiotics-treated group also had normal vaginal microflora with ample protective lactobacilli compared to women taking the placebo. This well-conducted study indicates that an appropriate orally administered probiotic can be effective in preventing BV. Together, the clinical studies show that use of some lactobacilli-based probiotics holds promise for the prevention and treatment of BV.

Recommendations for BV

- Pregnant women should regularly consume yogurt containing live cultures of *Lactobacillus acidophilus* to help prevent BV and consequent risk of premature delivery. This also may help prevent atopic eczema in the newborn (Chapter 7).

- Women who have BV or recurrent episodes of BV should take a *Lactobacillus* probiotic as well as a live-culture yogurt. The best use would be a probiotic containing hydrogen-peroxide-producing *Lactobacillus*.
- *Lactobacillus rhamnosus* GR-1 and *Lactobacillus fermentans* RC-14 are especially recommended.

CANDIDAL VAGINITIS

Frequently Asked Questions

What is candidal vaginitis?

Candidal vaginitis is a vaginal infection due to an overgrowth of a *Candida* species of yeast.

Is candidal vaginitis different than BV?

BV is caused by bacterial pathogens, while candidal vaginitis is caused by a species of yeast.

What are the symptoms of candidal vaginitis?

Most women with vaginitis due to candida experience itching, burning on urination, and a white discharge. It is important to get an accurate diagnosis so that effective treatments can be used.

How is candidal vaginitis treated?

Candidal vaginitis is treated with antifungal medications.

Can probiotics help in candidal vaginitis?

Probiotics may help in the prevention of candidal vaginitis.

Vaginitis caused by *Candida* species is second only to BV as a cause of vaginal infections, and it is one of the most common reasons for visits to a gynecologist.[15] Unlike BV, which is caused by bacterial pathogens, *Candida* are yeasts. *Candida albicans* is the yeast that causes the most vaginal infections, although other *Candida* species, such as *C. glabrata,* may be involved. Non-albicans *Candida* infections may be more persistent and difficult to treat, and are growing in frequency.[16] Risk factors for candidal vaginitis are pregnancy, therapy with antibiotics, use of oral contraceptives, diabetes, and intrauterine device (IUD) use.[17] Although the reason why some at risk get this infection and others do not is unknown. Almost all women experience a *Candida* yeast infection at some point in their lives, particularly after taking antibiotics. Antibiotic destruction of vaginal lactobacilli may predispose a woman to a yeast infection, but this has not been proven to cause candidal vaginitis.

Symptoms of a candida vaginal infection include itching, burning, and a thick, white discharge. Microscopic examination of the discharge or a vaginal swab reveals the presence of the characteristic yeast cells, usually with pseudohyphae (branching filaments) (see Figure 5.2). This is the diagnostic sign sufficient to confirm candidal vaginitis.

Antimicrobial Treatments for Candidal Vaginitis

In recent years, more effective oral antifungal (yeasts are fungi) medications have become available. Some, like fluconazole, are so

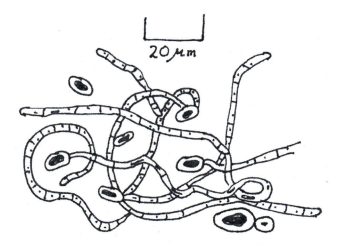

FIGURE 5.2. *Candida albicans* showing pseudohyphae (germ tubes). *Source:* Illustration by Lynne V. McFarland.

potent against *Candida albicans* that they can be given as a one-time dose to affect a cure. Effective topical antifungal creams—for example, miconazole or clotrimazole—vaginal tablets, and vaginal suppositories are available without a prescription. So why is there an interest in probiotics if conventional treatment is so easy? For reasons that are not understood, many women experience repetitive infections with *Candida*. Other women become infected with the more difficult-to-treat non-albicans species of *Candida* or strains of *Candida albicans* resistant to common antifungals. Preventing infection is the paramount goal. In particular, a probiotic that could decrease the associated risk of developing a yeast infection would be most welcome by women undergoing antibiotic therapy.

Probiotics and Candidal Vaginitis

Alternative treatments to conventional antifungal drugs have long been popular for vaginitis. In a survey at the Temple University Vaginitis Referral Center in Philadelphia,[15] 73 percent of patients had used over-the-counter antifungals, spending an average of $50 each, and 42 percent had used alternative medications. Of these, half had tried lactobacillus tablets, either orally or vaginally (11 percent), or yogurt, either orally (21 percent) or vaginally (18 percent). The median expenditure for these alternative treatments was $35. It is very important to realize that many yogurts are not prepared with strains of lactobacilli that have properties helpful for vaginitis. As discussed earlier, a probiotic microorganism for vaginitis should be ingestible orally, yet it should achieve effective concentrations in the vagina. It also should adhere to cells lining the vaginal tract, act against candidal infection, and stimulate the immune system to help eliminate the infection. Dairy strains of lactic acid bacteria used to make yogurt are not selected to have these properties. There is limited evidence that an appropriate *Lactobacillus* probiotic might be of some help in preventing vulvovaginal candidiasis.[16,17]

The same strain of lactobacilli probiotic taken orally has been recovered in the vagina,[12] presumably due to the proximity of the anal and vaginal orifices (see Figure 5.3).

One of the first controlled studies of the effectiveness of a probiotic yogurt for prevention of candidal vaginitis involved women in-

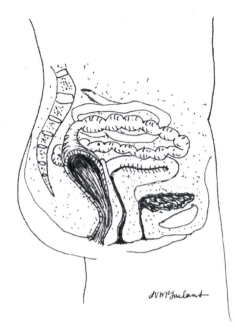

FIGURE 5.3. Proximity of portals of entry (anus, vagina, and urethra) used by microbes to gain entrance into the body. *Source:* Illustration by Lynne V. McFarland.

structed to take a special *Lactobacillus acidophilus* yogurt for six months.[18] The number of infections were recorded, and then the women were crossed over to the control treatment (no yogurt) for another six months. This strain of *Lactobacillus* was a good producer of hydrogen peroxide. The use of yogurt containing *Lactobacillus acidophilus* strain reduced the average number of candidal vaginal infections from 2.54 (no yogurt) to 0.38 (with yogurt). Although informative, this study does not provide strong evidence for the effectiveness of yogurt for candidiasis, since the dropout rate was high, with many women refusing to go on to the "no yogurt" phase of the study. In the end, only 13 of 33 women completed the entire crossover study. A later study by the same investigators treated women with recurrent candidal vaginitis with suppositories containing *Lactobacillus* GG. Subjective improvement was reported, but there was no placebo-control comparison group.[19] On the other hand, another group of investigators was unable to show a difference in candidal vaginitis with the use of a yogurt containing a hydrogen-peroxide-producing strain of *Lactobacillus acidophilus* as compared to a pasteurized yogurt control.[12] A decreased percentage of women with positive *Candida* cultures was observed in both the living and pasteurized yogurt groups. Their results may be explained by the nonviable pasteurized yogurt having an anti-*Candida* effect. For example, probiotic effects using heat-killed lactobacilli have been noted in immunodeficient mice.[20] As discussed earlier, BV incidence in this same study was lower in the live-culture yogurt group.[12] The probiotic yeast, *Saccharomyces boulardii,* has been shown to inhibit *Candida albicans* in germ-free mice, but studies in human candidiasis have not been reported.

Recently, results from a large placebo-controlled clinical trial for a mixture of *Lactobacillus* were published in a prominent medical journal. This study received considerable media attention and was touted as the "final answer" on the effectiveness of lactobacilli and vaginal candidiasis: that it does not work. The study enrolled 235 premenopausal women who received antibiotic therapy for an infection.[21] The women received one of the four possible treatments (*Lactobacillus* powder, *Lactobacillus* tablet, both the powder and a tablet, or placebos) during the time of antibiotic therapy and for four days afterward. The *Lactobacillus* product was described as containing *L. acidophilus* and *Bifidobacterium longum,* and the vaginal preparation as containing *L. rhamnosus, L. delbrueckii, L. acidophilus,* and *Streptococcus thermophilus.* Overall, 23 percent of the enrolled women developed a yeast infection, but there was no significant difference in the risk for developing an infection between the probiotics-treated women (26 percent) and the placebo group (17 percent). On the basis of this study, can we now say that lactobacilli probiotics are not effective in preventing vaginal candidal infections? Probably not, yet. Although the study examined a large number of women and was seemingly conducted carefully, it did not thoroughly describe the product being tested. There is no information whether the lactobacilli were hydrogen-peroxide-producing strains, whether they migrated to the vagina and adhered, or showed any other activities that would make these tested strains useful in preventing a yeast infection. The investigators stated that the product tested as containing viable lactobacilli as per the label, but the concentrations of live lactobacilli taken on a daily basis by the patients were not stated. As has been noted, further studies of ill-defined probiotics for candidiasis should be condemned.[16] Data from well-designed trials using defined products is needed so that an objective assessment of probiotics for vaginitis can be made.

Recommendations for Candidal Vaginitis

- Women who develop a *Candida* infection should take an appropriate antifungal medication to eradicate the yeast. The prescription drug, fluconazole, is an excellent treatment and is usually effective as a single, one-time dose. Over-the-counter antifungal creams such as miconazole and clotrimazole also can be effective.
- During the antifungal treatment and for seven days afterward, women with candidal vaginitis should consume about 4 oz of a good yogurt containing "live cultures" twice a day for 14 days. This regimen is nutritional, has no side effects, is inexpensive, and may help prevent yeast vaginitis. At this time, yogurt douches or probiotic capsules are not recommended because there is insufficient evidence of benefit. The oral yogurt recommendations are based on limited data; however, there is no harm and the treatment may even do some good.

URINARY TRACT INFECTIONS

Frequently Asked Questions

What are the symptoms of urinary tract infections (UTI)?

Most people experience burning on urination and have cloudy urine. They may also have lower-back pain.

What causes UTI?

Most UTI are caused by a bacterium called *Escherichia coli*.

How is UTI treated?

Antibiotics can effectively treat most UTI, but recurrences may necessitate frequent antibiotic use.

Can probiotics help in the case of UTI?

The jury is still out on the effectiveness of probiotics for UTI.

UTI are one of the most common forms of bacterial infection. Recurrences are frequent. A study in women who were followed-up after one UTI found that 42 percent had a recurrence within a year.[22] A gram-negative coliform (found in the human colon and feces) bacterium called *Escherichia coli* is the pathogen responsible for over 80 percent of infections in nonhospitalized women.[17] UTI occurs mainly in women, but may also occur in older men and those with abnormalities in their urinary tract or prostate. Sexual intercourse with a new partner or use of a diaphragm with spermicides increase the risk for UTI.[23] Symptoms include a burning sensation upon urination, painful voiding, and, sometimes, lower-back pain. Urine often is cloudy. Without prompt medical attention, the pathogen may infect the kidney (pyelonephritis), which is a more serious condition.

Nearly 25 percent of UTI cases will recur within a year.

Antimicrobial Treatments for UTI

The recommended treatment of uncomplicated UTI is a three-day course of trimethoprim/sulfamethoxazole. However, many patients cannot take sulfa drugs and pathogen resistance to trimethoprim/sulfamethoxazole is increasing, so a short course of a fluoroquinolone such as ciprofloxacin may be an option. Therapy with either antimicrobial treatment usually is successful. However, the pathogens may be more difficult to treat in hospital-acquired UTI cases. Recurrent UTI may involve long-term use of antimicrobials or continuous daily dosing to eradicate the pathogen and prevent further infection. Adverse effects with antibiotics and increasing pathogen resistance to antimicrobials through continued exposure make an alternative approach to prevent UTI recurrences highly desirable. Cranberry juice consumption is one such promising alternative.[24] Cranberry juice has been shown to block adhesion of *E. coli* to vaginal cells, and there is evidence that it can help prevent UTI recurrences. There also is interest in use of probiotics for UTI prevention.

Probiotics for UTI

Women with recurrent UTI have an increased propensity to have urinary pathogens colonize the vaginal tract.[25] Investigators at the University of Washington in Seattle showed that women with recurrent UTI had lower amounts of hydrogen-peroxide-producing lactobacilli in the vagina compared to healthy women who did not experience recurrent UTI.[26] The presence of *E. coli,* the pathogen involved in most UTI, also was associated with the absence of hydrogen-peroxide-producing lactobacilli. Thus, a rationale exists for probiotic use of lactobacilli, especially hydrogen-peroxide-producing strains that could colonize the vaginal tract and eliminate the source of *E. coli* and other UTI pathogens. However, it is difficult for orally administered lactobacilli to reach the vagina and adhere in sufficient concentrations to interfere with *E. coli.* Most clinical studies to test probiotics for UTI have involved instillation directly into the vagina or into the urethra. While these studies show some effectiveness of probiotics, the intravaginal or intraurethral dosing techniques do not seem practical in preventing UTI. An optimal probiotic microbe for UTI would have the same features as one for intestinal use: stimulation of a local immune response, production of pathogen inhibitory compounds, and inhibition of pathogen or pathogen action.

There have been only a few well-controlled investigations of probiotics for UTI, but those studies that have used microbial strains with desirable attributes for use in UTI show some promise. Investigators at the Lawson Research Institute in Toronto, Canada, have been most active in selecting optimal strains of lactobacilli for UTI.[27-29] They showed that the intravaginal insertion of specially selected lactobacillii reduced the incidence of recurrent UTI in a small group of high-risk women, but no controls were used for comparison.[29] In a later study, they compared the use of *Lactobacillus* vaginal suppositories with control suppositories for treating UTI recurrences following antibiotic treatment. The recurrence rate in the controls was 8 out of 17, compared to 3 out of 14 among those treated with the pro-biotic.[30] A larger placebo-controlled study (n = 47) in Norway did not find a therapeutic effect for a twice-weekly application of a commer-cial *Lactobacillus casei* (strain rhamnosus) (Gynophilus) vaginal suppository product in UTI-prone women.[31] There was no difference in the frequency of UTI in six months of follow-up nor were the lactobacilli found more frequently in the probiotics-treated women, suggesting that the *Lactobacillus* strain that was used did not adhere to urogenital cells and was not optimal for treating UTI. Another re-cent study showed there was a reduced recurrence of UTI in women taking cranberry-lingonberry juice compared to those who did not.[24] A third group took a *Lactobacillus*-GG-containing drink, but the con-sumption of this drink had no effect in preventing UTI. *Lactobacillus* GG is effective for intestinal disorders but has not shown any benefi-cial effect for vaginal or urinary infections.

More work is needed to establish the potential of probiotics for UTI. The practicality of frequent, long-term vaginal application of a probiotic is open to question. It would be highly desirable to establish that oral use of a probiotic reduces UTI recurrence rates.

Recommendations for UTI

- At the time of writing this book, the use of oral probiotics to treat or help prevent UTI is not recommended.
- There is some evidence for intravaginal use of selected probio-tics, but this technique seems impractical for daily use to prevent recurrent UTI.
- More evidence and testing of promising probiotic strains of lactobacilli are needed for a probiotic approach to help with UTI treatment and prevention.

SUMMARY

Of the randomized, controlled clinical trials that investigated pro-biotics for urogenital infections, the most promising results are for

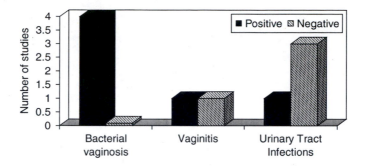

FIGURE 5.4. Number of randomized controlled trials showing effectiveness (positive studies) or no effect (negative studies) of probiotics compared to a control group for various genital and urinary tract infections.

the treatment and prevention of bacterial vaginosis (see Figure 5.4). More research should be directed at probiotic use for candidal vaginitis and urinary tract infections.

Chapter 6

Inflammatory Bowel Disease, Irritable Bowel Syndrome, and Digestive Problems

Many people suffer from distressing bowel and digestive conditions that persist for years or for their entire lifetime. The cause may be an infectious pathogen or an immune system problem, or may even be unknown. These digestive and bowel maladies can be extremely frustrating to treat and control. Probiotics offer a possible solution to some of these conditions.

CROHN'S DISEASE

Frequently Asked Questions

What is Crohn's disease?

Crohn's disease is a chronic, autoimmune, and an inflammatory condition involving the intestinal tract. Usually, the lower small intestine (ileum) and colon are the most affected organs. Symptoms of this disease include diarrhea, abdominal pain, and loss of appetite, but sometimes may be even more serious.

The Power of Probiotics
© 2007 by The Haworth Press, Inc. All rights reserved.
doi:10.1300/5597_06

What causes Crohn's disease?

The exact cause is unknown, but Crohn's disease is a malfunction of the immune system, possibly triggered by bacterial antigens.

How is it usually treated?

The usual line of treatment is diet modification, use of anti-inflammatory drugs, steroids, and, as a last resort, surgery.

Can probiotics help treat Crohn's disease?

Yes, new evidence indicates that probiotics can help treat Crohn's disease.

Crohn's disease is one of the two major inflammatory bowel diseases (IBD). The other is ulcerative colitis, which is discussed later. The two diseases are distinguished by the location of the inflammatory lesions and how deeply they penetrate the intestinal mucosa. Crohn's disease has more inflammatory involvement in the small intestine, although usually the colon is also involved. Crohn's disease lesions are deep and likely involve all the layers of the intestinal wall. The resulting thickening and swelling of the wall can cause intestinal obstruction, which can then be life threatening. Deep ulcerations and swelling of the lymph nodes in the area may develop. Affected areas of the small intestine may be dispersed with perfectly healthy sections, thus producing a "cobblestone" appearance. The disruption of the epithelial barrier may allow enteric (intestinal) bacteria to move from the intestine into the bloodstream. This "leaky gut" hypothesis explains how a disturbance of the microflora may incite the immune system to work overtime and cause inflammatory diseases such as Crohn's disease, ulcerative colitis, or irritable bowel syndrome.[1]

---

30 to 40 percent of people with Crohn's disease have at least two episodes per year

---

From the patient's perspective, it is abdominal pain, diarrhea, and intestinal cramps that usually prompt the first visit to the physician. Rectal bleeding may occur, as well as fever. Not surprisingly, loss of appetite and weight loss result from this spectrum of problems. Myriad extra intestinal signs and symptoms may be experienced by about one-third of Crohn's disease patients.[2] These include skin rashes and lesions, eye pain and vision difficulties, painful joints, jaundice, kidney stones, and gallstones.

A more serious potential complication of Crohn's disease is the blockage of the bowel, which inhibits or prevents defecation. Life-threatening complications associated with Crohn's disease are perforation of the intestine and toxic megacolon. With the latter, inflammation in the colon progresses to a point where there is little muscle tone and dilation begins. Without prompt treatment, the colon can burst and spill huge amounts of dangerous bacteria into the peritoneal cavity and bloodstream.

Unfortunately, the cause of Crohn's disease is not known; otherwise, more targeted treatments could be developed. In essence, something triggers the immune system to inappropriately activate itself and set up an inflammatory process in the digestive tract. Studies carried out in animal models of the disease have shown that the intestinal bacteria are important to the disease process. Rats and mice can be taken away from the mother at birth and raised in a sterile environment. These so-called germ-free animals have no microorganisms in or on their bodies. They do not develop Crohn's disease or ulcerative colitis. Triggers of Crohn's disease other than the resident bacteria also may exist, but are not yet understood.

Medications for Treatment of Crohn's Disease

Since the cause of the disease is not known, treatments are directed to alleviate the signs and symptoms of the disease. The core treatment of Crohn's disease involves anti-inflammatory agents delivered directly to the intestinal tract and this approach is certainly helpful. An ideal drug would be taken orally, would not be absorbed, and would obtain a high anti-inflammatory action only in the diseased regions of the digestive tract. While this ideal is elusive, existing drugs are cleverly designed to achieve some of these attributes. The basis for several of the better drugs is the local release of 5-aminosalicylic acid (5-ASA). 5-ASA is chemically and pharmacologically related to aspirin (acetylsalicylic acid). Sulfasalazine and olsalazine have no anti-inflammatory action per se, but upon exposure to the bacteria in the gut they are enzymatically hydrolyzed to release 5-ASA. Mesalamine is 5-ASA. It is usually formulated in a tablet or capsule that is coated so that it starts to dissolve and release the drug only after it reaches the intestine. Suppositories are another available dosage form. Mesalamine is a first-line drug for Crohn's disease, but is not without problems. Some 5-ASA is absorbed into the bloodstream, and those intolerant of aspirin will not be able to take mesalamine.

Antibiotics often are used in combination with other treatments because gut microorganisms often trigger intestinal inflammation.[3] The problem with this approach is that the bacteria responsible for setting off the disease process are not known. Antibiotics are a blunt sword that kill or suppress both good and bad bacteria, or fail to affect the disease initiator. Furthermore, repetitive or chronic use of antibiotics to treat this chronic disease results in resistance to antibiotics.

When Crohn's disease does not respond well to mesalamine and antibiotics, more powerful drugs may be needed. Unfortunately, there also may be increases in adverse effects. These medicines include steroids (often prednisone), immunosuppressive drugs (for example azathioprine, methotrexate, and cyclosporin), and a new monoclonal antibody known as infliximab, (marketed under the name Remicade). Infliximab is very expensive, costing thousands of dollars per year. Surgery is a treatment of last resort when drugs do not work.

Probiotics for Crohn's Disease

There has long been an interest in using probiotics for Crohn's disease, but until recently there were few controlled studies to carefully test whether probiotics would help. The results of the new studies show that probiotics offer a new approach to treating this debilitating disease. The rationale for probiotic use is, fundamentally, that the intestinal flora plays a role in the disease. As discussed earlier, the body's inappropriate response to bacteria in the gut seems to be involved. Normally the body does not mount an inflammatory immune response to indigenous bacteria. This is called immunological tolerance. However, in Crohn's disease and ulcerative colitis, the tolerance is lost and an inappropriate inflammatory response occurs. Given the complexity of more than 400 different bacteria in the intestines, it is not surprising that the specific resident bacteria involved in the inflammatory response are not known. Involvement of one or more transient pathogenic bacteria cannot be ruled out. In any event, it should be possible to modify the adverse microbial balance leading to the disease by use of an appropriate probiotic. Furthermore, some probiotics can enhance the immune response to certain antigens, especially to pathogen antigens,[4,5] and this effect could impact the disease favorably. Animal studies of IBD have demonstrated beneficial effects with probiotics.[6] For example, special strains of mice (IL-$10^{-/-}$) that spontaneously develop colitis do not develop colitis when raised in a germ-free condition. These germ-free mice are sterile; they have no bacteria at all. When they are brought into a nonsterile but pathogen-free environment, they rapidly develop intestinal disease. The disease process is much less severe when animals are pretreated with a *Lactobacillus plantarum* probiotic.[7] These results and the encouraging findings in other animal studies have prompted similar research in humans.

There now have been several controlled clinical trials of probiotics for Crohn's disease. The findings are summarized in Table 6.1. As we have pointed out, probiotic microorganisms differ in effectiveness for specific medical problems. *Lactobacillus* GG, which is well proven for benefit in pediatric diarrhea, seems ineffective for Crohn's disease. *Escherichia coli* Nissle 1917 was tested in one small trial, but was not found to provide a statistically significant benefit but only a benefit trend. A larger study is warranted to better understand the value of this probiotic for Crohn's disease. *Saccharomyces boulardii*, however, was shown to be helpful in two studies. While more research is needed, there is at least one probiotic that can be recommended for Crohn's disease.

It should be noted that the clinical studies evaluated the benefit after months of probiotic treatment and the doses of the probiotics tested were moderately high. The *E. coli* Nissle 1917 was used at a dose of 25 billion live bacteria given daily for one year. The *S. boulardii* dose was about ten billion living yeast given for two to six months (two capsules in the morning and evening every day). Other probiotic microorganisms also may be helpful for Crohn's disease, but there are no published studies to evaluate their effectiveness.

TABLE 6.1. Controlled clinical trials evaluating probiotics and Crohn's disease.

Probiotic	Number in study	Type of control	Result	Reference
Lactobacillus rhamnosus GG (LGG)	45	Placebo	10.5% recurrence in placebo 16.6% recurrence in LGG, ns	Note 8
Lactobacillus rhamnosus GG (LGG)	11	Placebo	50% relapse in LGG, ns 60% relapse in placebo	Note 9
Saccharomyces boulardii (Sb)	17	Placebo	4.6 stools per day at week 10 in placebo 3.3 stools per day at week 10 in Sb*	Note 10
Saccharomyces boulardii (Sb)	32	Mesalamine	38% relapse in mesalamine 6% relapse in mesalamine plus Sb*	Note 11
E. coli Nissle 1917 (Ec)	28	Prednisone	58% relapse in prednisone plus placebo 33% relapse in prednisone plus Ec, ns	Note 12

*Probiotic significantly better than control, $p < 0.05$, ns = probiotic not significantly different than control.

Recommendations for Crohn's Disease

- Conventional medicines should be used to induce remission of Crohn's disease.
- A probiotic should be used to help maintain remission.
- Saccharomyces boulardii has the best evidence for benefit.

ULCERATIVE COLITIS

Frequently Asked Questions

What is ulcerative colitis (UC)?

UC is a chronic inflammatory condition involving the colon. Symptoms include bloody diarrhea, abdominal pain, and loss of appetite. Symptoms may be severe.

What causes UC?

The exact cause of UC is unknown, but it is a malfunction of the immune system, possibly triggered by bacterial antigens.

How is UC usually treated?

The typical line of treatment is diet modification, use of anti-inflammatory drugs, steroids, and, as a last resort, surgery.

Can probiotics help treat UC?

Yes, new evidence indicates that probiotics can help treat UC.

Ulcerative colitis (UC) shares many similarities with Crohn's disease. Both diseases result in acute diarrhea, have a genetic predisposition, and are caused by the body's inappropriate response to the bacteria in the gut. Animal models clearly show that intestinal bacteria are needed to manifest these diseases. Laboratory animals that are used to study these diseases do not develop signs or symptoms when they are "germ-free;" that is, they have no bacteria.[13,14] In humans, these diseases attack those portions of the intestinal tract where the bacterial numbers are highest. Both diseases, in their severe form, can result in toxic megacolon with risk of perforation and spillage of dangerous intestinal microorganisms into the peritoneal cavity and bloodstream. Nevertheless, there are enough differences between Crohn's disease and UC to warrant classifying them separately. With Crohn's disease, inflammation involves the ileum and colon. Lesions usually are patchy with deep penetration of the intestinal tissue. UC involves only the colon, and has a continuous diffuse inflammatory appearance. The inflammation is on the mucosal surface without deep penetration. A hallmark of UC is bloody diarrhea, often accompanied by mucous and fever.[15,16]

Children tend to have more serious UC than adults

Medications for Treatment of UC

As with Crohn's disease, treatment is directed toward relief of symptoms rather than attacking the cause of the illness. Anti-inflammatory drugs and steroids are used to induce remission of the symptoms. Since the disease is confined to the colon, these drugs may effectively be given by enema or suppository. Mesalamine suppositories may be helpful, as are various oral delivery forms of 5-aminosalicylic acid (5-ASA) that release the drug only in the colon. With a more serious disease condition, high-dose oral or intravenous corticosteroids may be used. Immunosuppressive drugs such as azathioprine or cyclosporin may be used in a severe attack. Unlike in Crohn's disease, antibiotics and infliximab are rarely used for treatment of UC. Surgery to remove some or the entire colon is a treatment of last resort.

UC is associated with a higher risk of colon cancer

Probiotics for UC

Use of probiotics to attempt to restore the "normal" flora of the intestine seems logical because an imbalance of the intestinal microflora is involved in setting up the inflammation characteristic of both Crohn's disease and UC. Because of severe colonic inflammation, strong medications are needed to induce remission. Once the symptoms have subsided, the number of relapses in a fixed amount of time can be measured so that the effect of probiotic treatment can be compared to placebo or conventional drugs.

Probiotics have been tested for UC (see Table 6.2). The probiotic *E. coli* Nissle 1917 was found to be as effective as the standard treatment using mesalamine for UC.[17-19] This probiotic could be offered as an alternative to mesalamine for those patients intolerant of mesalamine or similar drugs. Of special interest would be a study examining the benefit of adding the probiotic to conventional mesalamine therapy to address whether probiotics should be combined with conventional treatments of UC. In two smaller "open" clinical trials (no placebo or other control group), *S. boulardii* and VSL#3 (a mixture of eight types of lactic-acid-producing bacteria) showed promise.[11,20] Controlled studies are needed before the extent of effectiveness can be determined.

The difference in relapse rates in the three studies using *E. coli* Nissle 1917 is most likely due to the different mesalamine doses and varying observation times. More study is needed on probiotic treat-

TABLE 6.2. Clinical trials evaluating probiotics and ulcerative colitis.

Probiotic	Number in the study	Type of control	Result	Reference
E. coli (Nissle 1917) (Ec)	116	Mesalamine	73% relapse in mesalamine 67% relapse in Ec, ns	Note 17
E. coli (Nissle 1917) (Ec)	103	Mesalamine	11% relapse in mesalamine 16% relapse in Ec, ns	Note 18
E. coli (Nissle 1917) (Ec)	327	Mesalamine	36% relapse in mesalamine 45% relapse in Ec, ns	Note 19
Saccharomyces boulardii (Sb)	24	None	17/24 had a successful outcome	Note 11
VSL#3 (mix)	20	None	15/20 had no relapse in 12 months	Note 20

ns = probiotic not significantly different than standard treatment.

ment of UC, but from what is already known, *E.coli* Nissle 1917 offers a reasonable alternative to mesalamine for treatment. *S. boulardii* and VSL#3 hold promise but more study is needed before they can be recommended for UC. All three probiotics have been well tolerated by patients. Other probiotic microorganisms also may be helpful for UC, but we have no published studies to evaluate them.

Recommendations for UC

- *E. coli* Nissle 1917 may be as effective as mesalamine in the treatment of UC. It can be tried as an alternative treatment.
- Other probiotics show promise, but need randomized controlled trials to prove their effectiveness.

POUCHITIS

Frequently Asked Questions

What is pouchitis?

Pouchitis is an inflammation of the "pouch" that serves the same function as the large intestine after the colon has been surgically removed.

What causes pouchitis?

Overgrowth of bacteria in the pouch causes inflammation.

How is it usually treated?

Antibiotics are the mainstay of treatment.

Can probiotics help treat pouchitis?

Yes, new evidence indicates that probiotics can help prevent flare ups of pouchitis.

Pouchitis may develop after the large intestine (colon) is removed due to disease, trauma, circulatory problems, or other chronic conditions. About 10 to 20 percent of the patients with ulcerative colitis (UC) develop so severe a disease that both the colon and rectum have to be removed surgically.[21] Most of the patients undergo a procedure called ileal pouch-anal anastomosis, in which the ileum is connected to the anus, forming an intestinal segment that, in effect, replaces the diseased colon. While this surgery is a cure for UC, there could be complications, the most common one being an inflammation of the pouch. About half of the patients experience an episode of pouchitis within ten years of surgery, and more than two-thirds of them have multiple attacks.[22] Fortunately, treatment with antibiotics is usually successful, although some patients develop a chronic condition that may require a complex and prolonged therapy.

30,000 to 45,000 people develop pouchitis every year in the United States.

Antimicrobial Treatments for Pouchitis

Metronidazole, ciprofloxacin, or other antibiotics are used to suppress the bacterial overgrowth causing the inflammation. Although patients usually respond well, some do not respond to the treatment or relapse once the antibiotic treatments are stopped. Unresponsive cases require more complex therapies, including use of some of the drugs used for UC. Antibiotics are not without adverse effects, and long exposure to these drugs results in resistance. There is a strong need for an alternative approach to prevent pouchitis.

Probiotics for Pouchitis

Since overgrowth or imbalance of the bacteria in the ileal pouch triggers the onset and maintenance of pouchitis, use of an appropriate probiotic to restore benign microflora or to prevent the imbalance in the first place seems logical. Recent clinical evidence strongly supports this approach (see Table 6.3).

VSL#3, an interesting probiotic blend (four strains of lactobacilli, three of Bifidobacteria, and one *Streptococcus salivarius* subspecies thermophilus), has been the best-investigated probiotic for pouchitis. Three separate placebo-controlled clinical trials of VSL#3 have been reported. The first study evaluated VSL#3 in preventing recurrence in patients who were in remission following antibiotic treatment.[22] The second study tested VSL#3 to prevent pouchitis after the initial surgery to create the ileal pouch.[23] The third study involved patients with severe disease but in remission following vigorous antibiotic treatment.[24] In addition, the enrolled patients previously had not responded to treatment, had multiple recurrences in the past year, or required continuous antibiotic treatment to control the disease. In all

TABLE 6.3. Controlled clinical trials evaluating probiotics and pouchitis.

Probiotic	Number in the study	Type of control	Result	Reference
VSL#3 (mix)	40	Placebo	3/20 (15%) relapsed on VSL#3* 20/20 (100%) relapsed on placebo	Note 22
VSL#3 (mix)	40	Placebo	2/20 (10%) had first episode on VSL#3* 8/20 (40%) had first episode on placebo	Note 23
VSL#3 (mix)	36	Placebo	3/20 (15%) relapsed on VSL#3* 9/16 (56%) relapsed on placebo	Note 24
Lactobacillus rhamnosus GG (LGG)	117	No probiotic	3/39 (7%) had first episode on LGG* 23/78 (29%) had first episode on nothing	Note 25

*Probiotic was significantly better than controls at $p < 0.05$.

three studies, the number of first episodes or relapses was consistently lower in the VSL#3-treated groups than in the placebo groups. Most impressive were the beneficial effects of VSL#3 in the third study involving patients with severe disease who did not respond well to the usual therapies. The doses used in these trials were relatively high (600 to 900 billion living bacterial cells per day), but without significant adverse effects. VSL#3 can be considered an effective agent to help prevent pouchitis.

A large clinical study in the Netherlands showed that *Lactobacillus rhamnosus* GG reduced the risk of developing pouchitis following the initial surgery.[25] However, this research project had one major weakness: the comparison control group consisted of patients receiving only conventional treatments prior to the start of the *Lactobacillus* GG study. These are called "historical controls." However, the characteristics of the treated and control groups were similar. First episodes of pouchitis were far fewer among those receiving *Lactobacillus* GG. This probiotic is promising as a preventative agent.

Recommendations for Pouchitis

- Conventional antibiotics should be used to induce remission of the disease.
- Probiotics should be used to help maintain remission.
- VSL#3 is recommended for prevention of pouchitis.
- *Lactobacillus* GG also appears to be effective, although it is not very well studied.

IRRITABLE BOWEL SYNDROME

Frequently Asked Questions

What is irritable bowel syndrome (IBS)?

IBS is a common disorder of the intestines that results in bowel pain, bloating, diarrhea or constipation, and gas.

What causes IBS?

This disorder is idiopathic (unknown cause). There usually are no obvious abnormalities in the structure or function of the digestive tract.

How is IBS treated?

Treatments generally are unsatisfactory. Alterations in diet and various drugs to treat symptoms are helpful for some.

Do probiotics help in IBS?

The results are mixed. *Lactobacillus plantarum* is the most promising probiotic for IBS.

IBS is a perplexing disorder that affects many people. Up to 20 percent of the people in the United States and Europe are estimated to have some symptoms of IBS. It may affect 14 to 24 percent of women and 5 to 19 percent of men in the United States and England.[26] The diagnosis of IBS is made by excluding known causes of diseases with similar symptoms: the patient has symptoms, but colonoscopic examination of the intestine reveals no apparent abnormality. The medical team must rule out infection, Crohn's disease, ulcerative colitis, cancer, and other causes for the described symptoms. There are no established markers to aid in the diagnosis. However, most IBS patients experience at least two of the following symptoms: abdominal pain relieved by defecation, passage of mucus, bloating, altered stool frequency, or altered stool form. Quality of life may be severely diminished for many patients with IBS. The search for the cause of IBS continues. Some IBS patients are lactose intolerant or have food allergies, but these problems may be only part of the reason for their illness.

Three times as many women have IBS as men

Medications for Treatment of IBS

Since the cause of IBS seems to be multifactorial, there is no standard treatment strategy. If allergies to certain foods can be identified, exclusion diets may be helpful. Some patients benefit from therapies that target emotional and mental health. Stress reduction and relaxation techniques benefit some of the patients. Medications that are used to relieve symptoms of IBS include antispasmodics, smooth muscle relaxants, antidiarrheals, and laxatives or high fiber diets to relieve constipation. Tricyclic antidepressants or SSRI drugs such as fluoxetine (Prozac) may help patients with some of the psychological aspects of IBS, but these drugs have other pharmacological attributes that may not be beneficial for some patients. Alosetron (Lotronex) is a special case. Because of its adverse effects, the drug was removed from the market in the United States. Recently, the Food and Drug Administration approved this drug only for female patients with severe diarrhea-dominant IBS who have failed conventional treatments. Constipation is a common side effect but ischemic colitis (shutdown of blood supply to the colon) represents a rare but very serious risk associated with alosetron.

There is limited evidence that nonabsorbable antibiotics can relieve gas and related symptoms,[27] which suggests that some IBS symptoms may be related to bacterial overgrowth in the upper intestine.[28] Therefore, therapy with probiotics has the potential to modulate and normalize the bacterial populations in the gut.

Probiotics for IBS

Limited studies have demonstrated promise for probiotics in the treatment of IBS. However, not all clinical trials have shown significant benefit. In part, the mixed results may be due to the diverse nature of IBS. There may be subpopulations of IBS patients who respond to probiotic treatment, but the treatment effect may not be seen clearly if the studies involve only a small numbers of patients. As shown in Table 6.4, clinical evaluations of several probiotic lactobacilli have been published.

Lactobacillus plantarum treatment did not improve IBS in a small crossover study conducted in the United Kingdom.[29] In this study, patients first received placebo for four weeks, followed by the probiotic. However, a lower dose of probiotic was used in this study when compared to two other studies[30,31] that found positive results with *Lactobacillus plantarum*. In another small crossover study,

TABLE 6.4. Probiotics for the treatment of irritable bowel syndrome.

Probiotic	Number in the study	Type of control	Result	Reference
Lactobacillus plantarum 299v	12	Crossover study	No benefit in symptom scores, 8.0 on Lactobacillus and 8.5 on placebo, at four weeks, ns	Note 29
Lactobacillus plantarum 299v	40	Placebo	19/20 (95%)* IBS resolved on Lactobacillus at four weeks 3/20 (15%) resolved on placebo	Note 30
Lactobacillus plantarum DSM9843	60	Placebo	36%* on Lactobacillus had less pain at four weeks 18% on placebo had less pain	Note 31
Lactobacillus GG (LGG)	24	Crossover study	No benefit for pain or bloating, ns	Note 32
VSL#3	25	Placebo	Less bloating on VSL#3 at eight weeks* but no other benefit	Note 33
VSL#3	42	None	Clinical improvement associated with bacterial changes in stools	Note 34
Lactobacillus plantarum LPO1 with Bifidobacterium breve BRO	50	Placebo	52% less pain and 44% less symptoms (probiotics) compared to 11% less pain and 8.5% less symptoms (placebo) at 28 days	Note 35
Bifidobacterium infantis	77	Placebo	Significant reduction in symptom scores compared with placebo and Lactobacillus salivarius	Note 36

*Probiotic significantly better than controls, $p < 0.05$.

ns = probiotic not significantly different than controls.

Lactobacillus GG was found to be not helpful,[32] but studies with VSL#3 and mixtures of *L. plantarum* and either *Bifidobacterium breve* or *L. acidophilus* decreased the symptoms as compared to placebo.[33-35] Another study compared self-reported IBS symptoms by patients treated with either *Lactobacillus salivarius, Bifidobacterium infantis,* or placebo.[36] The group treated with *B. infantis* reported improved symptom scores compared with placebo, but those treated with *L. salivarius* did not. These studies can be criticized for involving only a small number of patients and relying on patient's self-assessment for measuring outcomes. Nevertheless, probiotics show promise for treating IBS. The fact that other treatments are less than satisfactory for most IBS patients makes probiotic trials worthwhile, even though the evidence for efficacy is somewhat limited.

Recommendations for IBS

- Patients with IBS should consider using an appropriate probiotic as part of their treatment.
- *Lactobacillus plantarum, Bifidobacterium infantis,* and VSL#3 have the most evidence for usefulness to IBS.

LACTOSE INTOLERANCE

Frequently Asked Questions

What is lactose intolerance?

Lactose intolerance is a common digestive disorder resulting in cramps, bloating, diarrhea, and gas when lactose-containing foods or beverages are consumed.

Can probiotics help?

Theoretically yes, but no probiotic has been definitively shown to help. However, lactose-intolerant individuals usually may consume fermented milk products—for example, some yogurts—without problems.

Lactose intolerance is very common. It is estimated to occur, in about 75 percent of adults, less often in Europeans and more often in African Americans, Asians, and those of Mediterranean descent.[15,16] Lactose is a disaccharide (or sugar) that is made up of glucose and galactose linked together chemically. To split lactose for digestion, the body has an enzyme called lactase on the lining of the small intestine. People with lactose intolerance have low levels of this enzyme. The undigested lactose can cause diarrhea by creating a high osmotic pressure, which draws water into the intestine. And when undigested lactose reaches the colon, it may be fermented by the resident bacteria. The result is excessive gas, bloating, and diarrhea.

Medications for Lactose Intolerance

Milk and dairy products are the most common dietary sources of lactose. These can be avoided, but milk and dairy products are important sources of calcium and other valuable nutrients. Fat-free dairy products are beneficial. Lactose-reduced dairy products are now widely available and recommended for the lactose intolerant. Lactase tablets can be taken with foods containing lactose.

Probiotics for Lactose Intolerance

Yogurts and other fermented milk products may usually be consumed without problems by the lactose intolerant because the bacteria that carry out fermentation also make lactase. Thus, lactose in the milk product is reduced and some lactase is provided when the product is consumed. A person with lactose intolerance should purchase yogurts that are labeled as containing "live cultures." Bacteria that ferment these yogurts are added after milk pasteurization and retain the active enzyme. However, these yogurts may vary in the amount of lactose and lactase,[37] so those with lactose intolerance may want to try several brands to find the one that does not cause gastric distress.

Theoretically, consumption of a probiotic microorganism that contains high lactase concentrations and also adheres to the intestinal wall might provide enough lactase to digest food lactose. Such a probiotic (*Lactobacillus acidophilus* BG2FO4) was tested,[38] but unfortunately probiotic ingestion did not improve lactose intolerance in this clinical study.

Recommendations for Lactose Intolerance

- Fat-free or low-fat milk products are rich in calcium, protein, and other nutrients, and therefore should be a part of most diets. Those with lactose intolerance usually can tolerate "lactose-reduced" milk products or can consume the products together with lactase tablets.

- Most yogurts labeled as containing "live cultures" are an excellent source of nutrients, are low in lactose, and contain some lactase enzyme. These yogurts are recommended for the lactose intolerant.

CONSTIPATION

Frequently Asked Questions

Is constipation a common health problem?

Constipation is especially common in hospitalized patients, and chronic constipation is a common health problem among the elderly.

Is constipation serious?

Chronic constipation can adversely affect the quality of life. Severe constipation can lead to serious stool impaction.

How does fiber help?

Foods that contain indigestible fiber retain their bulk through the intestines, which facilitates intestinal transit and bowel movements.

Can probiotics help in constipation?

Limited evidence suggests that probiotic consumption may be helpful. Everyone experiences constipation from time to time, but the chronic constipation frequently experienced by the elderly or the incapacitated can be painful and demoralizing. If the stool becomes impacted, invasive medical procedures may be required for elimination. Impacted stools are a frequent problem in the bedridden elderly. Any disease that slows down the transit time of fecal material through the intestinal tract will increase the risk for chronic constipation. A diet low in indigestible bulk also will increase the chance for constipation.

Medications for Constipation

The best treatment for chronic constipation is to increase the bulk and water content of the stool so that elimination is facilitated naturally. High-fiber diets with ample fruits and vegetables are ideal. Bulking agents taken as supplements will accomplish the same (but without the valuable nutrients). Examples are bran, methylcellulose, polycarbophil, and psyllium. Wetting agents such as docusate allow the stool to pass easier. Osmotic agents such as lactulose and magnesium draw water into the stool and increase its bulk so that peristalsis (intestinal contractions) is increased. The use of stimulant laxatives is to be generally discouraged because they can have adverse effects and can be habit forming.

Probiotics for Constipation

Fecal bacteria play an indirect role in stool elimination. They act on foods reaching the colon and increase acidity. They also release metabolites that increase colonic osmotic pressure, drawing water into the stool environment. For example, metabolism of undigested disaccharides by the bacteria in the colon releases acetic acid and other low-molecular-weight fatty acids that stimulate intestinal mobility. Differences in the bowel bacteria between constipated and healthy subjects have been noted,[39] and so there is a rationale for increasing certain bacteria in the colon that might stimulate the transit time. However, few placebo-controlled studies exploring this approach have been published. Two recent studies demonstrate promise for the application of probiotics in constipation. A study in Finland involved 28 subjects from a nursing home.[40] Volunteers took a control juice or juice containing *Lactobacillus reuteri* or *Lactobacillus rhamnosus* and *Propionibacterium freudenreichii* for four weeks. A 24 percent increase in stool frequency compared to controls was observed in the group receiving the *Lactobacillus rhamnosus and Propionibacterium freudenreichii* juice. A second study was a well-designed clinical trial involving 70 adults in Germany with chronic constipation who were given a control beverage or a probiotic beverage containing *Lactobacillus casei* Shirota for four weeks.[41] The probiotic group experienced significantly less constipation by several criteria and increased stool frequency. Probiotic use was needed for a week before

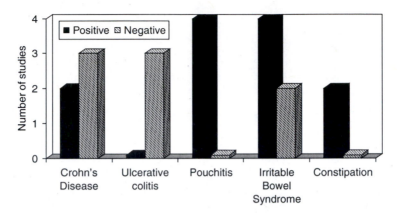

FIGURE 6.1. Number of positive and negative randomized controlled trials with probiotics for various types of inflammatory bowel diseases or constipation.

improvement was evident. While more studies are needed, probiotics hold promise for helping relieve constipation.

Recommendations for Constipation

- With few adverse effects, probiotics are worthy of a trial for chronic constipation. However, it may take several weeks for improvements to be noticed.
- A probiotic containing *Lactobacillus casei* Shirota is especially recommended.

SUMMARY

For digestive diseases that involve the immune system, probiotics seem to offer an effective therapy for some conditions but not for others (see Figure 6.1). Pouchitis, irritable bowel syndrome, and constipation have more supportive studies than negative ones. In contrast, Crohn's disease and inflammatory bowel disease are not as well supported by positive studies.

Chapter 7

Allergies

Allergies are sharply increasing in the developed countries. It is estimated that 20 percent of the population in the developed countries suffer from allergies,[1] whereas allergies are not as prevalent in the developing countries. Probiotics may be useful in moderating the immune response to various antigens involved in allergies.

The most common types of allergic diseases are hay fever, asthma, eczema, contact dermatitis, food allergies, and hives. These types of allergic diseases are an inappropriate response by the immune system to different antigens (compounds that cause antibody production). Allergies are often seen during infancy as a skin rash, which may be associated with consumption of a particular food or in response to environmental factors. The common term for this skin rash is *eczema,* but it is more appropriately termed *atopic dermatitis* (if it is not due to a known skin irritant such as diaper rash or poison ivy). Atopy is due to hypersensitivity to environmental allergens and is genetically determined. Infants with atopic dermatitis, as they grow older, are at a higher risk for developing allergic rhinitis (hay fever) and asthma. An acute asthma attack can be life threatening, and chronic asthma often necessitates continuous and complex drug therapies to manage the disease.

The Power of Probiotics
© 2007 by The Haworth Press, Inc. All rights reserved.
doi:10.1300/5597_07

Most common antigens that cause allergies:

- Pollens
- Molds
- Dust mites
- Animal dander
- Insects
- Food (nuts)
- Medications

What could be the cause of the rapid increase in allergies over the past few decades? Some people blame the increasing environmental pollution and others blame modern lifestyle changes. Unfortunately, the cause simply is not known. One intriguing hypothesis is the "hygiene hypothesis." This hypothesis may explain how probiotics might help in alleviating allergies. The hygiene hypothesis, outlined in London in 1989,[2] may explain some of the soaring rates of allergies in those populations with high living standards.[3] The hypothesis is based on the belief that stimulation of the immune system by the intestinal microorganisms or from infections at birth and during infancy is important for its healthy maturation. At birth, a newborn has no microbial microflora in his or her intestines. Rapidly, the baby picks up microorganisms from the mother and the environment. In a superclean environment, the microbes that are acquired may not be ideal for stimulation of immune function. Birth by cesarean section in a hospital facilitates colonization by hospital microorganisms, which may not be appropriate. In contrast, home birth in a large household would facilitate acquisition of a very different set of microorganisms. Those born into a lower socioeconomic household or in a developing country may be rapidly exposed to a diverse microbial population. The same environmental factors influence the composition of a nursing mother's microbial flora and, hence, what she would pass on to her infant. The use of antimicrobials and vaccines reduce infections and hence the immune stimulation involved in normal childhood diseases. This is not to advocate the limiting of vaccine use, but it is likely that the childhood illnesses prior to the era of vaccines and antibiotics were strong stimulants to the immune system.

One in five people in the developed countries has allergies

Evidence to support the hygiene hypothesis comes from many sources. Comparative studies of allergic dermatitis or asthma in first-born children and children born in small, affluent families to those born into large families show an increased asthma risk for children in less crowded households.[2,4,5] The microbial flora of infants with allergies has been shown to differ from that of nonallergic infants. Higher numbers of clostridia and staphylococci have been seen in infants with allergic dermatitis, whereas the healthy controls had higher numbers of bifidobacteria in their stools.[6,7] Swedish children living in communities where little antibiotic and vaccine use along with high lactobacilli intake in dairy products is the norm had lower rates of atopic allergies than those living in a more conventional setting.[8,9]

A history of infections also has been correlated with allergic reactions. Evidence of a previous infection with hepatitis A, *Toxoplasma gondii,* and *Helicobacter pylori* was associated with a lower incidence of airway allergies in Italian and U.S. subjects.[10,11] If natural infections and rapid acquisition of lactic-acid-predominant intestinal microflora at birth protect against the development of allergy, one can appreciate the interest and potential of introducing beneficial microbes early in life. Limited evidence indicates that probiotic use has the potential to help decrease allergies that are becoming more common in Western countries. This chapter focuses on the use of probiotics for infantile allergic dermatitis because the strongest evidence for probiotic efficacy rests here, and an infant with atopic dermatitis is at risk for developing respiratory allergy and asthma later in life. The limited evidence for beneficial probiotic effects in adults will be briefly considered.

ATOPIC DERMATITIS (ECZEMA)

Frequently Asked Questions

What is atopic dermatitis?

Atopic dermatitis is a hypersensitivity to food or other environmental antigens that results in a rash. It often is called eczema.

Is atopic dermatitis related to hay fever and asthma?

Atopic dermatitis usually manifests itself in infancy, while hay fever or asthma usually follow later in childhood and in adulthood. All three are allergic manifestations resulting from an inappropriate response of the body to substances in the environment.

What causes atopic dermatitis?

The tendency to develop atopic dermatitis is inherited, but not everybody whose parents have allergies will develop atopic dermatitis. Other factors, yet to be determined, also play a role.

How is atopic dermatitis treated?

Steroid creams can help reduce inflammation and itching. Stronger anti-inflammatory drugs also may be needed.

How can atopic dermatitis be prevented?

Special diets that eliminate suspected food allergens can help, so also the removal of precipitating agents in the environment.

Can the use of probiotics help with atopic dermatitis?

One of the most exciting new applications for probiotics is to help reduce atopic dermatitis and other allergies.

Atopic dermatitis can be defined as a genetically determined hypersensitivity to environmental chemicals, foods, and other allergens. It is associated with a family history of allergies and often is manifest during the first few months of infancy. When one parent is affected by atopic allergies, there is a 50 percent chance that the infant will also be affected. When both parents are affected, the probability that their child will develop allergies increases to more than 80 percent.[12] Infants with atopic dermatitis frequently experience allergic rhinitis (sometimes called hay fever) and asthma as they get older. The atopic dermatitis rash may appear, along with itching, on the face, eyelids, scalp, or diaper area,[13] as shown in Figure 7.1. Development of sensitivity to common household chemicals and fragrances is frequent.

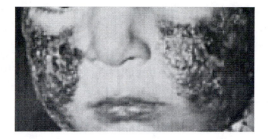

FIGURE 7.1. Picture of a severe case of eczema. *Source:* Courtesy of National Library of Medicine.

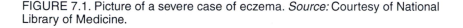

Atopic patients frequently become allergic to particular foods (most commonly, nuts) and show a positive skin test to many common allergens. Not all rashes are atopic in nature—some rashes simply may be an inflammatory response to contact with an irritant, such as a dirty diaper or laundry detergent residues. In infancy, an atopic rash consists of weeping, crusted patches called eczema. The rash appears and then disappears, but scratching the involved areas aggravates the inflammation, which may then lead to an infection.

Topical Treatments for Atopic Dermatitis

If the offending allergen can be identified, then avoidance is optimal. However, hypersensitivity to multiple and unidentified agents often makes total avoidance of the allergen impractical and ineffective. Over-the-counter topical hydrocortisone creams can provide some relief from itching and reduce inflammation. However, long-term use of these creams is not recommended because it can lead to thinning of the skin and systemic effects in infants. Older antihistamines may relieve itching but are sedating. Newer nonsedating antihistamines do not seem as effective in relieving itching. Moisturizing skin creams are helpful. In severe cases, short courses of oral steroids may be needed. A new approach of using prescription ointments containing immunosuppressive drugs (tacrolimus and pimecrolimus) has been successful for some, but there is concern about the long-term effects of immunosuppressants on the skin.

Probiotics for Atopic Dermatitis

How would ingestion of a probiotic microorganism influence allergic reactions in skin and airways? This solution, at first, may seem implausible and not likely to succeed. However, clinical evidence shows that there is a benefit in both prevention and treatment of atopic allergies. The mechanistic explanation for the beneficial effects of probiotics in atopic dermatitis, atopic rhinitis, and asthma may lie in the validity of the hygiene hypothesis that was discussed earlier. This hypothesis proposes that an infant born into a small, affluent family may not get full exposure to a wide variety of microorganisms that are involved in appropriately stimulating the immune system. Without acquiring a full spectrum of microbes, the infant is not well adapted to respond to environmental antigens that will be encountered later in life. Also, the use of antibiotics during childhood may perturb the healthy balanced microbial flora needed for immune stimulation. An ultraclean household limits the microbial and antigen exposure during this time of the infant's immune system development. The probiotic approach provides a beneficial microorganism that will help stimulate an "antiallergenic" immune response. Ideally, this is done at birth so that early allergic reactions can be prevented. Probiotics have been used to successfully treat atopic dermatitis in infants. Microbial flora dominated by bifidobacteria and lactobacilli lowers the risk of developing atopic allergies in infants.[7] Clinical studies have exclusively tested the strains of these two types of probiotics. Research has shown that there are several possible mechanisms of probiotic action that may explain their beneficial effects for allergic patients. The best-studied probiotic microorganism in this regard is *Lactobacillus rhamnosus* GG. *Lactobacillus* GG has been shown to degrade and partially digest a common antigenic protein found in milk (casein).[14,15] Once partially digested, the milk protein has a lesser ability to activate a T-cell response (a type of immune regulatory cell), which is characteristic of an allergic response. However, it is not known whether a similar digestion takes place in the human gut when the *Lactobacillus* probiotic is ingested.

Probiotics also may be effective for allergies because they can change the levels of different types of cells involved in the body's immune response, such as antibodies and immune helper cells (T-cells). *Saccharomyces boulardii,*[16] *Lactobacillus* GG,[17] and other probiotics[18] stimulate the production of IgA antibodies in the intestinal tract. These IgA antibodies bind antigens and keep them from being absorbed. Since IgE antibodies also are involved in the allergic response, probiotics may work by modulating IgE levels. Also, the ability to increase T helper 1 (Th-1) cells and decrease T helper 2 (Th-2) cells may be important.[19] Th-1 lymphocytes are involved in cellular immunity and oppose the involvement of Th-2 cells in allergic reactions. Production of Interleukin-10, believed to protect against allergic responses, is enhanced in atopic children treated with *Lactobacillus* GG.[20] Evidence of decreased antigen absorption in infants with cow's milk allergy and atopic dermatitis and of reduced intestinal inflammation is also associated with *Lactobacillus* GG use.[21]

Clinical evidence for the efficacy of probiotics for atopic dermatitis is summarized in Table 7.1. Six of the seven studies used *Lactobacillus* GG, a probiotic that can survive in the human intestinal tract. Five studies involved probiotic treatments for infants or children who had atopic dermatitis. These studies show that this probiotic can successfully treat existing atopic dermatitis, although the responses generally were not complete resolution of disease. One study evaluated a heat-killed *Lactobacillus* GG, as well as a living *Lactobacillus* GG preparation, both being compared to an indistinguishable placebo.[23] Unexpectedly, 5 of the 13 patients experienced diarrhea and were prematurely terminated from the study. Breaking the treatment assignment code revealed that all the adverse effects were in the heat-killed *Lactobacillus* GG group. The outcome of this study was measured using SCORAD which is a scoring system to describe, in a quantitative way, the severity of atopic eczema. The decrease in SCORAD scores was greatest in the viable *Lactobacillus* GG group and was significantly different from placebo. These findings suggest that living probiotic microorganisms are best to treat atopic dermatitis, and use of low-viability products, such as the killed probiotic preparation, may cause adverse effects.

A very important evaluation of a probiotic to prevent atopic disease was conducted in Turku, Finland,[26] and another report of the four-year follow-up also was published.[27] In this double-blind, placebo-controlled study, *Lactobacillus* GG or placebo was given to expectant mothers who had atopic dermatitis, allergic rhinitis or asthma, or a family history of atopic disease for two to four weeks prior to deliv-

TABLE 7.1. Probiotic studies for atopic dermatitis (AD).

Probiotic	Dose form	Population studied	Duration	Result*	Reference
Lactobacillus rhamnosus GG (LGG)	In formula	27 infants with AD and cow's milk allergy	1 month	SCORAD score = 15 in LGG, 19 in placebo	Note 21
Lactobacillus rhamnosus GG (LGG)	Capsules given to mother	10 nursing infants with AD	1 month	SCORAD score = 26 at start and 11 after one month	Note 21
Lactobacillus rhamnosus GG (LGG) or *Bifidobacterium lactis* Bb-12 (BI)	In formula	27 infants with AD	2 months	SCORAD score =1 in LGG, 0 in BI and 13.4 in placebo	Note 22
Lactobacillus rhamnosus GG (LGG) versus killed LGG	In formula	35 infants with AD	7.5 weeks	SCORAD score = 19 at start and 5 at end in LGG, 15 at start and 7 at end in killed LGG, and 13 at start and 8 at end in placebo	Note 23
Mix of *Lactobacillus rhamnosus* and *L. reuteri*	Powder to be added to a drink	43 children 1-13 years old with AD	6 weeks on probiotic, 6 weeks on placebo	56% improved in probiotic group, and 15% in controls	Note 24
Lactobacillus rhamnosus GG (LGG)	Given to mothers only	62 mother-infant pairs	During pregnancy and lactation	In two years, 47% infants in placebo group developed eczema versus only 15% in LGG group	Note 25
Lactobacillus rhamnosus GG (LGG)	Capsules to mothers, powder in liquid to infants	132 healthy mother-infant pairs with family history of atopic disease	Starting 2 months before delivery and continued for 6 months to infants or to mothers if breast-feeding	Eczema in 23% probiotic group and 46% placebo at age 2; in 26% in probiotic group versus 46% at age 4	Note 26,27

*p < 0.05, probiotic was significantly better than the placebo.

A decrease in the SCORAD score indicates improvement.

138

ery. In this setting, the infants would be at a high risk of developing atopic disease. Following delivery, the mother continued to take the probiotic for six months if she was breast-feeding; if she was not breastfeeding, the infant was given the probiotic directly for six months. Atopic dermatitis was reduced by half, compared to placebo, at both the two-year and four-year follow-ups for the child-mother pairs who received *Lactobacillus* GG. Also noteworthy is that the breast-feeding mothers taking the probiotic were able to pass on protection from subsequent disease to the infant who never directly received the probiotic. A subsequent examination of the subset of breast-feeding mothers showed that the breast milk levels of transforming growth factor β2, which is considered a marker of anti-inflammatory activity, were higher in those receiving *Lactobacillus* GG than those receiving placebo.[25] The breast milk of the mothers taking the probiotic indirectly provided the infant with some protection from the high risk of developing atopic disease. The fact that this protection lasted up to four years, even though the probiotic ingestion stopped at six months, shows that the impact on the infant immune system was early and long lived. It will be of great interest to monitor the children in later years to see if probiotic exposure in the first weeks of life provides the protection against allergic rhinitis and asthma, which typically develop at an older age.

Recommendations for Atopic Dermatitis

- The most important application of a probiotic in atopic diseases is to prevent the disease from starting in infancy. Expectant mothers who have atopic diseases (atopic dermatitis, allergic rhinitis, or asthma), or a family history of atopic disease, or a father with a family history of atopic disease, should begin taking an effective probiotic two to three months before the expected delivery date and continue for at least six months after the delivery.
- The mother should take the probiotic until the infant is weaned.
- Probiotic treatment of atopic dermatitis in an infant should be started as soon as possible and continued for at least two months. The probiotic powder can be mixed with juice or water.
- *Lactobacillus rhamnosus* GG is the probiotic with the best evidence for efficacy in treating and preventing atopic dermatitis. At

the time of writing this book, it is not known whether probiotic use will effectively prevent or treat allergic rhinitis or asthma later in life.

ADULT ALLERGIES

Human clinical studies to evaluate the effectiveness of probiotics for allergies have almost exclusively involved infants, with the goal of determining whether probiotics can prevent or relieve atopic dermatitis (eczema). One assumption is that, if atopic dermatitis can be prevented in infancy, the risk of allergic rhinitis and asthma may be decreased in adulthood. This has not been proven, but it seems reasonable. As previously discussed, probiotic administration can favorably influence immune response. For example, *Lactobacillus rhamnosus* GG increased antibody titers against rotavirus in children[28] and *Bifidobacterium lactis* HN019 increased aspects of cellular immunity in elderly volunteers.[29,30]

Yogurt generally is fermented from milk using cultures of *Lactobacillus bulgaricus* and *Streptococcus thermophilus*. An early study of live-culture yogurt given to atopic adults showed no beneficial immunological effects, but the yogurt was given for only one month.[31] However, a one-year study conducted at the University of California, Davis, gave encouraging results for the potential of probiotics to decrease adult allergies.[32] Investigators set up the study to measure the responses of a young, healthy group (age 20 to 40 years) and a senior group (age 50 to 70 years) to a one-year consumption of live-culture yogurt (Dannon). To control for calcium and the effects of other dairy nutrients, a control group received heat-inactivated yogurt. Another control group received no yogurt at all. The number of days of allergic symptoms in both the young and senior populations decreased significantly in the live-culture yogurt group compared to the controls. The total IgE, an antibody type associated with allergic reactions, was lower in the senior group that consumed the live cultures. There was a difference in the pattern of allergic response between the young and the senior groups. In those receiving the live-culture yogurt, a sharp decrease in the total number of days of allergies was noted at the three-month assessment of the young group, whereas the decrease was slower to manifest in the senior group. This may be due

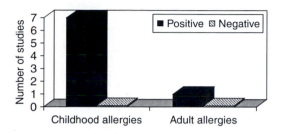

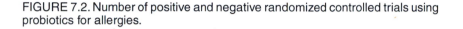

FIGURE 7.2. Number of positive and negative randomized controlled trials using probiotics for allergies.

to the slower immune responsiveness of older adults. It is noteworthy that the study did not select the adults suffering from allergies, and so the outcome of reduced allergic symptoms by yogurt was unexpected.

As shown in Figure 7.2, all six studies performed with children and one with adult patients found probiotics to be effective for reducing allergic reactions. More studies are needed but the results to date show promise for the use of probiotics for allergies. Future research should use a specific probiotic known to have strong effects on the immune system (for example, *Lactobacillus rhamnosus* GG) and test the probiotic in an allergic population for at least one year, and then the potential of the probiotic approach for allergy relief can be better assessed.

Recommendation for Adult Allergies

- Adults suffering from allergies should consume at least 8 oz of live-culture yogurt per day. This provides an excellent source of calcium and other micronutrients, and may provide some relief from allergies.

Chapter 8

Miscellaneous Disorders

Advertisements for many dietary supplements sold in the United States, Europe, and Asia often include diverse health or beauty claims. Sometimes the claims seem too good to be true. In this chapter, we discuss the evidence that support or do not support the use of probiotics for a number of miscellaneous disorders that are not covered in the other chapters.

Probiotics are living organisms that have complex interactions with other microbes and biological functions. In recent years, research has shown that probiotics produce a wide variety of substances that have diverse pharmacological actions. For example, short-chain fatty acids are formed in the human intestine by bacterial fermentation of fiber. These short-chain fatty acids have anti-inflammatory effects, reduce insulin production, and improve lipid metabolism. Some probiotic strains are efficient producers of short-chain fatty acids. This is one of the many reasons that probiotics can be effective for a wide variety of diseases. In this chapter, the evidence for a miscellaneous array of claimed uses for probiotics will be discussed.

The Power of Probiotics
© 2007 by The Haworth Press, Inc. All rights reserved.
doi:10.1300/5597_08

RHEUMATOID ARTHRITIS

Frequently Asked Questions

What is rheumatoid arthritis?

Rheumatoid arthritis is an autoimmune inflammation of the joints that is often triggered by an infection and a subsequent overreaction of the immune system.

How can probiotics have an effect on arthritis?

Probiotics can help break down foods or other substances that inappropriately stimulate the immune system.

Can probiotics help treat rheumatoid arthritis?

More clinical trials are needed, but early results show some promise.

Why would a probiotic help against a disease that is thought to be a result of degenerative changes in the joints? There are two major types of arthritis—osteoarthritis and rheumatoid arthritis. Osteoarthritis usually involves the weight-bearing joints. Typically, the cartilage is worn out by chronic use and a bony overgrowth leads to loss of functioning (see Figure 8.1). This type of arthritis is more common in the elderly. Probiotics have not been tested for osteoarthritis.

Rheumatoid arthritis can strike at any age. It differs from osteoarthritis, which is caused by an inflammatory reaction that produces a buildup of immune complexes in the synovial fluid and synovium (lining of the joint) that results in stiffness of the joints. Rheumatoid arthritis may develop after an infection, such as intestinal infections caused by *Salmonella typhimurium, Shigella, Campylobacter,* and *Clostridium difficile.* If parts of the bacterial cell wall find their way into the small blood vessels near the joints, the immune system becomes very active in an effort to clear this bacterial debris from where it does not belong. The influx of immune cells into this narrow area causes swelling and damage. Probiotics may help relieve this type of arthritis.

An early clue that dietary components may be involved in rheumatoid arthritis came from the studies using simple diets. Liquid elemen-

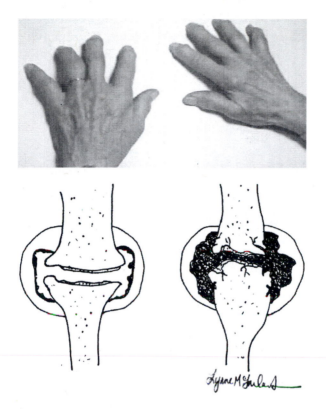

FIGURE 8.1. Different types of arthritis are shown. The photograph at the top is an example of rheumatoid arthritis. On the bottom left is shown osteoarthritis, which is characterized by thin cartilage and bone spurs where no cartilage protects the bone. The synovial fluid (black) is mildly inflamed. On the bottom right is rheumatoid arthritis, which is an autoimmune disease that initially attacks the synovium (lining of the joint), causing inflammation (black) and degradation of the bone with time. *Source:* Photograph and illustration by Lynne V. McFarland.

tal peptide diets were found to decrease the symptoms of rheumatoid arthritis, hypothetically due to less antigenic (proteins) stimulation of the immune system. One theory holds that a disrupted intestinal microflora cannot break down food proteins well, leading to a hyperactive immune response to the large undigested proteins. Because probiotics help in both digestion and immune system functioning, they may have a role in reducing the immune overreaction seen in rheumatoid arthritis. In one study, mice prone to develop arthritis were given *Lactobacillus casei* strain Shirota. These did not develop arthritis, in contrast to mice that were given a placebo.[1]

Two clinical studies of probiotics in humans with rheumatoid arthritis gave conflicting results. One study randomized 43 patients with rheumatoid arthritis to a vegan diet (no animal products of any kind) rich in lactobacilli (the strains were not described) or a control diet (not containing lactobacilli) for one month.[2] Arthritis symptoms significantly improved in the group given lactobacilli. However, a second study did not confirm this finding. This small study randomized 21 people with rheumatoid arthritis to *Lactobacillus rhamnosus* GG (four capsules per day) or placebo for one year.[3] No differences in the number of tender or swollen joints or other measurements of arthritis were seen in the two groups. There have been no published studies with probiotics in people with osteoarthritis.

Recommendation for Rheumatoid Arthritis

- More clinical trials are needed to ascertain if probiotics can be helpful for rheumatoid arthritis.

CANCER

Frequently Asked Questions

How can probiotics have an effect on cancer?

Some cancers result from exposure to carcinogenic (cancer-causing) substances in food or in the air. Probiotics may reduce the concentration of intestinal enzymes that convert precancerous substances to carcinogenic compounds.

Can probiotics help prevent cancer?

Not all types of cancer can be helped by probiotics, but there is some evidence that probiotics may be useful for the prevention of bladder and cervical cancers.

A health claim for probiotics, reported in several review articles, is prevention of some forms of cancer.[4,5] Historically, different countries have extremely different risks for developing certain types of cancers, and it was first thought that this was due to diet. Later research determined that it was not directly due to diet itself or genetic differences, but the risk for some cancers may be explained, in part, by different metabolic activities in the intestinal microbial flora. When people at high risk of colon cancer (Japanese living in Hawaii) were compared to people at low risk (rural Japanese and Africans), distinct differences in their normal flora were seen.[6] If the differences in intestinal microflora could affect cancer risk, how can probiotics help prevent cancer? One way is that certain probiotic bacteria (*Lactobacillus acidophilus, Bifidobacterium bifidum,* and *Enterococcus faecalis*) can bind proteins in foods that can cause mutations (mutagens) that may lead to cancer. Once bound by the probiotic, mutagens cannot be absorbed from the intestine and transported to other parts of the body and are thus excreted harmlessly. Another mechanism by which probiotics may prevent cancer is to interfere with production of enzymes that in turn produce carcinogens. Precarcinogens can be present in food (azo dyes, pesticide residues, or compounds in burned meat) and are changed by enzymes produced by the normal intestinal flora to active carcinogens, which may result in colon or other types of cancer. Levels of some of these enzymes are reduced when some probiotics are given to humans. Probiotics also have been shown to reduce the size and recurrence of some tumors in mice. All this indirect evidence has convinced researchers to initiate clinical trials to test probiotics for the prevention of cancer.

Several clinical trials have investigated the protective role of microflora and the prevention of recurrences of cancer in humans (see Table 8.1). A *L. casei* strain decreased the recurrences of bladder cancer in two studies. Twenty-three patients with a history of bladder cancer were given oral *L. casei* (3 g/day) and 25 were not given any.[7] Patients who were given lactobacilli had a significantly longer period before their bladder cancer recurred (mean of 350 days) compared to control patients (195 days, $p = 0.03$), and no adverse reactions were noted. A second randomized study using the same *L. casei* probiotic was conducted in 125 patients with bladder cancer.[8] Patients with primary multiple or recurrent single tumors who were given the *Lacto-*

TABLE 8.1. Randomized controlled trials testing probiotics for the prevention of cancer.

Population	Probiotic tested	Dose of the probiotic	Recurrence of cancer in groups	Reference
48 adults with bladder cancer	Lactobacillus casei	3 g/day	57% in probiotic group and significantly more (83%) in controls ($p < 0.05$)	Note 7
125 with bladder cancer	Lactobacillus casei	3 g/day	20% in probiotic group and significantly more (46%) in controls ($p < 0.05$)	Note 8
228 women with cervical cancer	Lactobacillus casei LC9018	Not given	Enhanced tumor suppression, better survival in probiotic group, exact data not given ($p < 0.05$)	Note 9
61 women with cervical cancer	Lactobacillus casei LC9018	Not given	Significant tumor reduction ($p < 0.05$)	Note 10

bacillus had fewer recurrences of bladder cancer, but there were no significant differences compared to controls when patients had recurrent multiple tumors. The probiotic *Lactobacillus casei* LC9018, a strain of bacteria that reduced tumor size in animal studies, was tested in a randomized trial of 61 patients with cervical cancer who were receiving radiation treatments.[10] Patients receiving LC9018 had significant reductions in tumors compared to control patients receiving radiation alone. In a follow-up study, 228 patients with cervical cancer were randomized to *L. casei* LC9018 or placebo, and more tumor regression was noted in the probiotic group.[9]

Although there is indirect evidence that the intestinal flora or ingested microbial agents may be involved in the prevention of other types of cancers, the direct evidence is limited. Additional controlled trials are needed in which patients are given the probiotics orally and then followed-up for cancer development.

Recommendations for Cancer

- More clinical trials are needed to establish the effectiveness of probiotics for bladder or cervical cancer.

- Because colon cancer is associated with exposure to dietary carcinogens, probiotics might be useful against this type of cancer
too, but randomized clinical trials are needed to demonstrate
benefit.
- Given the lack of risk associated with *Lactobacillus casei*, patients with bladder or cervical cancer might consider taking this
probiotic to help prevent recurrences. The patient should first
discuss this with his or her oncologist.

HIGH CHOLESTEROL

Frequently Asked Questions

How can probiotics have an effect on reducing cholesterol?

Probiotics can help increase cardiovascular health by directly bind-
ing cholesterol or influencing the metabolism of cholesterol by other
bacteria living in the gut.

Can probiotics help reduce high cholesterol?

Yes, but the effect is modest.
Cardiovascular disease is a leading cause of global mortality. In
the year 2000, cardiovascular disease accounted for 16.7 million
deaths worldwide. In the United States, half a million women die every year from heart attacks and stroke. Serum cholesterol levels (total
cholesterol, low-density lipoprotein [LDL], high-density lipoprotein
[HDL], and triglycerides) are highly correlated with ischemic heart
disease (low blood flow), stroke, and peripheral arterial disease. A
person with high total cholesterol, high triglycerides, high LDL, and
low HDL is at high risk for cardiovascular disease.
Probiotics frequently are credited for reducing cholesterol levels.[4]
Probiotics may act on cholesterol levels in two main ways. Probiotics
can inhibit those enzymes involved in making cholesterol in the body
or can bind dietary cholesterol and interfere with absorption from the
intestine. Then the dietary cholesterol is excreted along with the probiotic from the body without being absorbed and making its way into
the circulatory system.

	Desirable level (mg/dl)	Undesirable level (mg/dl)
Total cholesterol	<200	≥240
LDL	<100	≥190
HDL	>40	<40
Triglycerides	<150	>170

A review examined six randomized studies using a probiotic yogurt (two strains of *Streptococcus thermophilus* and one of *Enterococcus faecium*) for four to eight weeks versus control pasteurized yogurts to lower cholesterol levels.[11] The probiotic yogurt resulted in an average of 4 percent decrease in total cholesterol and 5 percent decrease in LDL cholesterol. Another review of 13 clinical studies showed 7 out of 13 (54 percent) of the trials found a significant difference between probiotic and control groups. The average was a 7 percent reduction in total cholesterol levels for people treated with various types of yogurts containing viable microbes.[12] For this book, we reviewed more than 20 clinical studies comparing various probiotics with controls for the reduction of cholesterol. Half the studies found a reduction in cholesterol levels, with the decrease ranging from 0.4 to 8 percent, and half of them did not find a significant reduction in cholesterol levels. By and large, the trials that did not show a significant reduction were conducted with healthy volunteers who had nearly normal cholesterol levels. Restricting the analysis to seven controlled trials in patients with higher-than-normal cholesterol levels, most of the trials showed a significant reduction in cholesterol levels for the probiotics-treated patients compared to controls (see Table 8.2). A reminder: High levels of total cholesterol, LDL cholesterol, and triglycerides increase the risk for heart disease and stroke. High levels of HDL cholesterol decrease the risk.

Clinical trials studying lipid levels have shown reductions in total cholesterol levels or LDL cholesterol, but some trials have shown no effect on HDL. In an open study with no control group, *Lactobacillus sporogenes* (4×10^8/day) was given for three months to 17 patients with hyperlipidemia. Total cholesterol levels fell from 330 to 226 mg/dl and LDL levels dropped from 267 to 173 mg/dl. There was no significant effect on HDL or triglyceride levels.[20] Without a comparison group, it cannot be concluded that the decrease was solely due to the probiotic. Two of three studies that did use a control group to compare with volunteers taking a probiotic found a significant reduction in both total cholesterol and LDL in the group taking a probiotic yogurt or a mixture of probiotic strains (Table 8.2).[13-15] It should be noted that when kefir (a fermented milk product) was tested, there

TABLE 8.2. Summary of randomized trials using probiotics for the reduction of cholesterol in patients with hypercholesteremia.

Population	Probiotic tested	Dose and duration of treatments	Reduction in the probiotic group from enrollment* (%)	Reduction in the control group (%)	Reference
40 adults with TC > 290 mg/dl	*Lactobacillus acidophilus* L1 yogurt	200 g/day in yoghurt for four weeks	TC: −3.2** LDL: −4.1**	TC: +0.3 LDL: −0.2	Note 13
32 adults with mild to moderate hypercholesteremia	*Enterococcus faecium* and two strains of *Streptococcus thermophilus*	200 g/day for eight weeks	TC: −5.3** LDL: −6.1** HDL: no change	No change in placebo	Note 14
13 adults with TC > 232 mg/dl	Kefir product (mixed strains)	500 ml/day for four weeks	TC: +0.7 ns LDL: +0.4 ns HDL: +0.9 ns	TC: −1.3 LDL: −2.6 HDL: +1.0	Note 15
324 adults with TC > 230 mg/dl	Red-yeast-fermented rice	1.2 g/day for eight weeks	TC: −23** LDL: −31** Trig: −34** HDL: +20**	No change in placebo	Note 16
83 adults with TC > 250 mg/dl	Red-yeast-fermented rice	2.4 g/day for eight weeks	TC: −17** LDL: −22** Trig: −11** HDL: 0 ns	TC: −0.3 LDL: −0.4 Trig: −0.6 HDL: 0	Note 17
14 adults with high cholesterol and HIV infection	Red-yeast-fermented rice (Cholestin)	2.4 g/day for eight weeks	TC: −30.8 mg/dl** LDL: −32.3 mg/dl** HDL: no change Trig: no change	No change in placebo	Note 18
50 adults with coronary heart disease	Xuezhikang, a cholestin extract	1.2 g/d for six weeks	TC: −20** LDL: −34** Trig: −32** HDL: +18**	No change in placebo	Note 19

*TC = total cholesterol; LDL = low-density lipoprotein; HDL = high-density lipoprotein; Trig = triglyceride; ns = not significant.

**Significantly reduced compared to controls, $p < 0.05$.

was no difference in the change of cholesterol levels between the treated group and the control group.[15]

Another probiotic, the red yeast, *Monascus purpureus,* had garnered its share of attention. This red yeast has been used for centuries in China as a food coloring and a rice-fermented food to increase blood circulation and improve cardiovascular health. Statin drugs, such as lovastatin, are very effective in reducing cholesterol and triglyceride levels by inhibiting an enzyme (HMG CoA reductase) involved in cholesterol production. Red yeast produces ten different types of monacolins (lovastatin having the highest concentration), all of which help to lower cholesterol levels. Red yeast is sold as a dietary supplement in the United States by a number of companies.[16-20] A dose of 2.4 g of most brands of red yeast is equivalent to 9.6 mg of total statins and 7.2 mg of lovastatin. The usual starting dose of the pharmaceutical drug, lovastatin, is 10 to 20 mg per day. Four randomized clinical trials found red yeast probiotics to be effective in reducing total cholesterol, LDL, and triglycerides when compared to placebo.[16-19] Reduction in lipid levels in the red yeast groups was substantial. For example, a 10 to 23 percent decrease in total cholesterol was achieved. In contrast, studies using other probiotics have shown only a mild reduction (< 8 percent) of total cholesterol.[21] However, every 1 percent reduction in cholesterol levels is associated with a 2 to 3 percent reduction in risk for cardiovascular heart disease, so even mild reductions may be important.[13]

Recommendations for High Cholesterol

- More clinical trials are needed to see whether probiotics are effective for abnormal blood lipids, but most studies show promising results. There are good drugs available that lower cholesterol levels, but they must be monitored for long-term effects on liver and muscle function.
- Long-term studies are needed to determine whether reductions in cholesterol levels that are seen in short-duration probiotic studies (6-8 weeks) persist over time.
- *Enterococcus faecium* and *Lactobacillus acidiophilus* are two of the most promising single-agent probiotics.

- Taking red yeast probiotics is essentially like taking a mixture of prescription statin drugs. The effects are powerful and most likely beneficial, but a physician should be consulted before initiating this therapy.
- The role of probiotics such as red rice yeast may be most beneficial for people who have slightly elevated cholesterol but have not yet developed any cardiovascular disease. However, clinical studies are needed to test this role. Statin drugs have beneficial effects other than just improving lipid profiles.

DENTAL HEALTH

Frequently Asked Questions

How can probiotics have an effect on dental health?

Bacteria in the mouth cause cavities. Some probiotics can decrease the number of these cavity-producing bacteria.

Can probiotics help for better dental health?

Probiotic may help for better dental health.

Few studies have tested probiotics for infections of the mouth, even though it is heavily populated by microflora, especially if gingivitis (infection of the gums) is present. Evidence that probiotics may be helpful in reducing cavities has come from studies using *Lactobacillus rhamnosus* GG (see Table 8.3). This probiotic produces a substance that inhibits the growth of *Streptococcus mutans,* a bacterium involved in cavity development. Long-term (seven months) consumption of milk containing *Lactobacillus rhamnosus* GG has been shown to reduce caries in day care children.[22] When two *Lactobacillus rhamnosus* strains were added to cheese and fed to young adults for three weeks, many of them had decreased counts of *Streptococcus mutans* by the end of follow-up (three weeks after treatment stopped) as compared to adults given control cheese.[23] In this study, there was no difference in counts of caries-causing bacteria during the three weeks of cheese intervention, showing that it perhaps takes

TABLE 8.3. Probiotics for the prevention of caries from randomized controlled trials.

Probiotic	Given to	Dose and duration	Effect in the probiotic group*	Effect in the control group	Reference
Lactobacillus rhamnosus GG in milk	594 children (1-6 years) in day care centers	Seven months	Risk of caries OR = 0.6, $p = 0.01$		Note 22
Lactobacillus rhamnosus GG and Lactobacillus rhamnosus Lr LC705 in cheese	74 adults (18-35 years old)	LGG (1.4×10^9/day) Lr LC705 (9×10^8/day) for three weeks	Streptococcus mutans count decreased in 8 out of 38 (21%) $p = 0.04$	Streptococcus mutans count decreased in 2 out of 36 (6%)	Note 23

*OR = odds ratio, a measure of the risk of caries. An OR below 1 denotes that the probiotic is effective in preventing the occurrence of caries if $p < 0.05$. For example, an OR of 0.5 means half the risk, whereas an OR = 2.0 means twice the risk.

time for the probiotic strains to colonize the mouth before inhibition of the bacteria can begin.

In the United States, 184 million cavities occur every year

Another study using a mixture of Lactobacillus strains, not including the strain *Lactobacillus rhamnosus,* was unable to demonstrate a probiotic-induced decrease in *Streptococcus mutans* levels in the mouth.[24] It may be that these strains do not produce the same inhibitory substance as *Lactobacillus rhamnosus*. Once again, optimum probiotic strain selection is critical for effective therapy.

Recommendations for Dental Health

- The two trials testing *Lactobacillus rhamnosus* for dental health show promising results, but more studies are needed before routine long-term use to prevent cavities can be recommended.
- More types of probiotics should be tested for dental cavity prevention.

DIABETES

Frequently Asked Questions

How can probiotics have an effect on diabetes?

Some probiotics can decrease insulin resistance in cells.

Can probiotics help for diabetes?

This is not known. Only animal studies and in vitro tests show promising results. No clinical trials have been reported.

There are 18.2 million people in the United States with diabetes, and the prevalence of diabetes on a global scale is rapidly increasing. Diabetes is associated with high health care use and costs. Complications of diabetes include retinopathy (blindness), neuropathy (loss of nerve sensation in the extremities), cardiovascular disease, and kidney disease. Although there are medications for diabetes, many people do not maintain good control of their blood glucose levels and hence develop these complications over time.

There has been some interesting research showing that *Lactobacillus casei* may have an influence on diabetes. Children with diabetes in Russia were treated with a strain of *Lactobacillus casei* (Acylact).[25] Probiotic treatment restored their normal microflora and stimulated their immune system (both are known effects of probiotics). The children also showed an unexpected decrease in hyperglycemia (high blood sugar). How could this happen? Diabetes can result when the pancreas stops producing insulin (type 1 diabetes) or when cells become resistant to insulin (type 2 diabetes). Insulin helps glucose to enter cells so that glucose can be used as an energy source. If glucose cannot be absorbed into the cells, it remains in the blood and causes problems. One of the most common early symptoms of diabetes is fatigue, which is associated with the loss of energy production. The body tries to get rid of excess glucose in the blood by increasing urine output, which leads to the other common symptoms of diabetes such as increased thirst, frequent urination, and unexpected weight loss. *Lactobacillus casei* produces substances that decrease insulin resistance by the cells, which may explain how this probiotic can improve the control of diabetes.[25,26] Unfortunately, no controlled clinical trials in humans have been performed to date, so this remains just a hypothesis.

Recommendation for Diabetes

- Human clinical studies are needed to determine if probiotics can be of help in the control of diabetes.

HEPATIC ENCEPHALOPATHY

Frequently Asked Questions

How can probiotics have an effect on hepatic encephalopathy?

Hepatic encephalopathy (liver disease) results from abnormally high blood levels of the breakdown products from proteins, especially ammonia. Some probiotics may metabolize these harmful products and clear them from the body.

Can probiotics help prevent or cure hepatic encephalopathy?

Initial results of probiotic trials show promise.

There have been claims that probiotics may be useful for patients with hepatic encephalopathy, a type of liver disease.[27] Patients with hepatic encephalopathy have an altered intestinal microflora, with increased concentrations of *Escherichia coli* and *Staphylococcus* species. This alteration and the reduction of the normal ammonia-metabolizing bacteria limits the clearance of this toxic compound from the intestines.[28] Only two clinical studies and three case series have been reported, with a total of 122 people studied.[28-30] A recent study of 55 adults with hepatic encephalopathy randomized patients to a probiotic mixture (*Pediacoccus pentoseceus, Leuconostoc mesenteroides, Lactobacillus paracasei,* and *Lactobacillus plantarum* 2592) or a placebo control group for 30 days. Significantly more patients (50 percent) given the probiotic mixture had resolution of their symptoms compared to the placebo group (13 percent).[28] In addition, serum ammonia levels dropped by 36 percent in the probiotic group compared to only 3 percent in the placebo group ($p < 0.05$). This study confirmed the earlier controlled trial that tested *Enterococcus faecium* SF68 against lactulose (a standard treatment).[29] There was a

50 percent reduction of serum ammonia levels in the probiotic group compared to no reduction in the control group.

Recommendations for Hepatic Encephalopathy

- The few studies that have been conducted show promise for probiotics for hepatic encephalopathy, but more clinical trials are needed.
- Either *Enterococcus faecium* SF68 or a specially tested mixture of probiotics is a good candidate for further testing.

HOSPITAL INFECTIONS

Frequently Asked Questions

How can probiotics have an effect on hospital-acquired infections?

Hospital workers and patients can carry disease-causing bacteria and transmit them to others. Probiotic use may reduce the carriage rate in both hospital workers and patients.

Can probiotics help prevent hospital infections?

Probiotics show promise, but further work is needed.

Hospital workers (nurses, physicians, and staff) and patients can harbor pathogenic microbes in many body sites, including the intestinal tract and nasal passages. Bacteria living in the nose are easily transmitted to patients and other staff members and may cause disease. Of most concern are microbes that can cause large outbreaks of disease in hospitals, such as *Clostridium difficile* or methicillin-resistant *Staphylococcus aureus* (MRSA). The latter is a highly dangerous antibiotic-resistant pathogen. Probiotics can compete with these pathogens for attachment sites or nutrients and displace them. Control of hospital infections traditionally has relied on infection control practices and the use of antibiotics, but the emergence of antibiotic-resistant strains of bacteria has caused concern over how these types of infections are treated. Recently, the use of probiotics has been investigated as a method to prevent these types of dangerous infections in hospitals.[31]

In one study, 209 volunteers were randomly given a probiotic milk drink containing *Lactobacillus rhamnosus* GG, *Bifidobacterium* B420, *Lactobacillus acidophilus* 145, and *Streptococcus thermophilus* or a standard yogurt as a control for three weeks.[32] At the beginning of the trial, 68 percent of the volunteers harbored potential pathogens. Among those given the probiotic mix, significantly fewer (55 percent) were carrying pathogens by the end of the study. No change was seen in the controls given yogurt containing no probiotics.

In a second study of 90 patients in an intensive care unit, patients were given either a probiotic mixture (*Lactobacillus acidophilus* La5, *Bifidobacterium lactis* Bb12, *Streptococcus thermophilus,* and *Lactobacillus bulgaricus*) or placebo for one week.[33] Of those given the probiotic mixture, significantly fewer (43 percent) harbored pathogens compared to those given placebo (75 percent). No side effects were seen in either study for those given the probiotic mixtures.

Recommendations for Hospital Infections

- Probiotics may offer a safe and an inexpensive method to reduce the frequency of nosocomial (hospital) outbreaks, but more clinical trials are needed before specific recommendations can be made.

HYPERTENSION (HIGH BLOOD PRESSURE)

Frequently Asked Questions

How can probiotics have an effect on hypertension?

Probiotics can lower leptin levels in the blood, which is involved in regulating blood pressure.

Can probiotics help in reducing high blood pressure?

Probiotics show promise.

Probiotics can indirectly affect blood pressure. Use can decrease tissue resistance to insulin (see the section on diabetes), which is associated with lower blood concentrations of leptin, which is involved in both fat metabolism and the modulation of blood pressure. Probiotics that can lower leptin levels in the blood would help reduce blood pressure. There have been several small studies showing a lowering of blood pressure in patients given probiotics.[11,34,35] For example, 36 healthy volunteers were randomized to *Lactobacillus plantarum* 299v (2×10^{10} cfu/day) or placebo.[34] After six weeks, blood pressure in the probiotic group fell from an average of 134 to 121 mmHg (a drop of 13 points), whereas those given the placebo went only from an average of 128 to 126 mmHg ($p = 0.001$). No adverse effects were reported. A study in Japan tested, in elderly hypertensive patients, milk fermented with *Lactobacillus helveticus* and *Saccharomyces cerevisiae*.[35] A small but significant decrease in systolic and diastolic blood pressure was seen in the fermented milk group compared to the group receiving a nonfermented milk.

It is estimated that one billion people will have high blood pressure by the year 2025

Recommendations for Hypertension

- Since hypertension is a very serious medical problem and there are excellent antihypertensive drugs that are available, more studies are needed before probiotics can be recommended.

IMMUNITY

Frequently Asked Questions

How can probiotics have an effect on immunity?

Microbes in the gut are involved in the stimulation of the immune system. Ingestion of certain probiotics may further stimulate immunity.

Can probiotics help stimulate immunity?

Yes, but further research is needed on the medical applications for this probiotic effect.

Microorganisms in the intestinal tract interact with the host at many different levels. It was recognized early on that microbiologically sterile (germ-free) mice are highly susceptible to an overwhelming infection if they are exposed to a pathogen. Once these mice are allowed to pick up normal intestinal flora, they become more resistant to infections. The reasons that the microbial flora help resist unwanted growth of pathogens are many, but an important one is the ability of the gut microbes to stimulate the immune system. The gut-associated lymphatic tissue (GALT) is the largest mass of lymphoid tissue in the body and is extremely important in immunological defense. The GALT is heavily influenced by intestinal microbes. IgA antibodies are secreted by the intestinal mucosa. These antibodies bind to toxins, allergens, and pathogens and keep them from translocating (moving) from the colon to the bloodstream. Also important is the role of intestinal microbes in stimulating immune responses in other parts of the body, mainly through production of nonspecific protective molecules by white blood cells. For example, researchers in New Zealand showed that an elderly group of volunteers receiving supplements of the probiotic *Bifidobacterium lactis* HN019 had increased amounts of blood leucocytes, and the ability of these white blood cells to phagocytose (ingest) a test bacterium improved.[36] Increases in natural killer cells (NK cells) and certain other types of protective blood cells were noted.

Of great medical interest is whether immune stimulation by ingestion of a probiotic can have practical benefits in preventing or ameliorating illnesses. The ability to mount a strong immune response declines with age, and therefore there are potential benefits of enhancing the immunity in older populations. Newborns and HIV-infected patients also have suboptimal immunological protection. Despite the well-documented increases in immune parameters among study subjects who were given probiotics,[36-39] there have been few studies measuring the resulting general health benefits.

A one-year study of yogurt consumption by 42 adults living in California showed intriguing results. Subjects received either live-culture yogurt, heat-killed yogurt, or no yogurt. Those receiving live-culture yogurt showed a decrease in allergic symptoms compared to subject receiving no yogurt.[40] In senior adults (> 55 years), there was a slight trend toward decreased gastric distress in the group consuming the live-culture yogurt, and there was a similar mild trend for decreases in colds and coughs. A larger study is needed to define the extent of protection by the yogurt. A study conducted in Italy used milk fermented with *Lactobacillus casei* DN-114001 or with normal yogurt cultures. There was a significant reduction (20 percent) in the duration of winter-type illnesses in the *L. casei* group. However, there was no difference in the number (incidence) of winter infections that developed in the two groups.[41] As nonprobiotic lactobacilli strains may also stimulate immune responses, the choice of a living-bacteria treatment as a control may have masked the protective effect of the *L.casei* strain in this study. A better control would have been a heat-killed yogurt.

As previously discussed, probiotics can increase specific IgA responses to viral infections. For example, *Lactobacillus rhamnosus* GG increased antibody titers against rotavirus in children[42] and *Saccharomyces boulardii* increased IgA antibody titers against pathogenic *Clostridium difficile*.[43] Indeed, probiotic action against pathogenic bacteria may depend, in part, on its ability to stimulate immune responses. What is still unclear is whether probiotics taken regularly will improve overall health by increasing immune function. It seems logical that probiotic use would be beneficial, but evidence to date does not conclusively prove it. Further research is urgently needed to measure illnesses in large populations of those taking or not taking an appropriate probiotic for an extended period of time. Measuring all infections and other illnesses in elderly population with probiotic use compared to a placebo group would be illuminating.

Recommendations for Weakened Immunity

- Daily consumption of a live-culture, quality yogurt is worthwhile. Yogurt is an excellent source of calcium and other nutrients. In addition, regular consumption of yogurt potentially may decrease allergies and improve immunity.
- Evidence is lacking to date as to whether regular use of specific probiotic microbial products will enhance immunity and result in better health.

SEXUAL DYSFUNCTION

Frequently Asked Questions

How can probiotics have an effect on sexual dysfunction?

Probiotics only indirectly have an effect on sexual dysfunction by increasing health and well-being.

Can probiotics help in sexual problems?

Despite some marketing claims, there is no direct evidence that probiotics have an effect on sexual dysfunction.

Although there are some who claim that probiotic use enhances sexual enjoyment, there are no scientific studies with probiotics that have targeted sexual dysfunction, nor do any of the probiotic mechanisms directly lend themselves to correcting this type of condition. Be suspicious of probiotics that claim to enhance sexual functions.

Recommendations for Sexual Dysfunction

- Before any clinical trials are performed, some basic research is required to show how probiotics might help in sexual dysfunction.

STOMACH ULCERS

Frequently Asked Questions

How can probiotics have an effect on stomach ulcers?

Probiotics may act on the bacterium that causes most stomach ulcers.

Can probiotics help in peptic (stomach) ulcers?

Yes, they can.

Stomach ulcers are commonly caused by a bacterium called *Helicobacter pylori*. Infection by this organism causes duodenal or stomach ulcers, heartburn, and gastric distress, and may increase the risk for gastric cancer. Contrary to popular belief, peptic ulcers are just as common in women as in men. The usual treatment using three oral antimicrobial medications helps ulcers heal, but may not eradicate all the *H. pylori* organisms colonizing the stomach lining, and it is often accompanied by deleterious side effects. These adverse effects include diarrhea, nausea, bloating, and taste disturbances. The effects can be so severe that people stop taking the antibiotics, leading to recurrence of the stomach ulcers.

---

15 to 20 percent of patients with peptic ulcers have bleeding ulcers

---

Several studies have tested the ability of probiotics to inhibit colonization of the stomach by *H. pylori* or supress the adverse effects of antibiotics. Only some probiotic strains seem to work for this condition. In animal models and laboratory tests, *Lactobacillus salivarius* and *L. acidophilus* inhibited the growth of *H. pylori*, but strains of *L. casei* did not.[44] In mice, *L. salivarius* also reduced inflammation associated with *H. pylori* infections. A number of human studies have been completed. A review of 13 clinical trials with various probiotics (*L. acidophilus, L. johnsonii, L. gasseri,* lactobacillus fermented yogurt, or *Bifidobacterium 15 longum*) found that 11 trials (85 percent) reported a reduction in *H. pylori* or the symptoms of antibiotic treatments.[45] Our review of the literature found 13 out of 15 clinical trials showed fewer adverse effects of antibiotic treatments or quicker times to ulcer healing. All the trials involved various strains of lactobacilli or bifidobacteria.

There were four randomized control trials testing probiotics for peptic ulcers. Three of the four showed that probiotics decreased symptoms or colonization rates of *H. pylori* (see Table 8.4). One study enrolled 60 adults colonized with *H. pylori* but without current symptoms.[45] All the adults were given the typical triple antibiotic treatment, but one group also received *Lactobacillus rhamnosus* GG (1.2×10^{10}/day) for 14 days, while the rest were given a placebo. The

TABLE 8.4. Probiotics studies for the reduction of *Helicobacter pylori* (stomach ulcers).

Probiotic	Population studied	Dose per day and duration	Result	Reference
Lactobacillus rhamnosus GG	60 asymptomatic carriers adults with triple antibiotic treatment	1.2×10^{10}/day, for 14 days	Less nausea and diarrhea (side effects of antibiotics) with LGG versus controls*	Note 44
Lactobacillus acidophilus La5 or Bifidobacterium lactis Bb12	70 asymptomatic adult carriers	2×10^7/ day or placebo milk, for six weeks	Significantly reduced H. pylori with Bifido-bacterium but not with Lactobacillus*	Note 46
Lactobacillus casei Shirota	20 asymptomatic adult carriers	3×10^8/day, for three weeks	Decreased H. pylori 64% in probiotic group versus 33% controls**, ns	Note 47
Lactobacillus johnsonii La1 or Lactobacillus paracasei ST11	326 asymptomatic children	Dose not stated for four weeks	L. johnsonii La1 affected 8% reduc-tion in H. pylori*,**	Note 48

*p < 0.05, probiotic had a significant effect compared to controls.

**Concentration of H. pylori measured by ^{13}C-urea hydrogen test.

group given the *L. rhamnosus* GG probiotic reported significantly fewer ($p < 0.05$) adverse effects than the placebo group, including taste disturbance (23 versus 50 percent, respectively), nausea (10 versus 37 percent, respectively), and diarrhea (3 versus 27 percent, respectively). Another small study showed a trend for reduction of *H. pylori* after three weeks of treatment with *L. casei* Shirota, but the difference between the probiotic group and the controls was not significant.[47] Lactobacilli probiotics may have an effective role in controlling colonization by *H. pylori,* but it would be of great interest to evaluate the effect of the probiotic treatment in patients with active stomach ulcers.

A survey of schoolchildren in Chile showed frequent asymptomatic carriage of *H. pylori*. One study enrolled 326 children, who were then randomized into one of five groups. Two types of probiotics (*Lactobacillus johnsonii* La1 or *Lactobacillus paracasei* ST11) were given as either a living preparation or a heat-killed preparation. One group of children received a placebo with no lactobacilli (either living or dead). After four weeks, only the children given the living *L. johnsonii* La1 probiotic had significantly reduced levels of *H. pylori*.[48] This study not only showed the value of one strain of probiotic but also showed that the probiotic should be living. In regions where *H. pylori* frequently occur, long-term administration of this probiotic strain may prove to be valuable in preventing future cases of stomach ulcers.

Recommendations for Stomach Ulcers

- Several strains of lactobacilli show promise in treating peptic ulcers and reducing the adverse effects associated with antibiotic treatments.
- *Lactobacillus* probiotics together with antibiotics should be used to help treat stomach ulcers.

STRESS

Frequently Asked Questions

How can stress have an effect on my health?

Studies have shown that stress can trigger the production of substances that stimulate your immune system, change the shape of cells lining your intestines, and affect the normal microbes living in your intestines.

How can probiotics have an effect on stress?

There is some evidence that probiotics can help correct the imbalances in your intestines' microbial flora that have changed due to stress.

Psychological or metabolic stress brought on by daily life, travel, or illness affecs the body in many ways. Stress has been shown to trigger allergic reactions in the intestines, which are involved in food intolerance and chronic inflammatory bowel conditions such as inflammatory bowel disease, ulcerative colitis, and colitis.[49] Stress can reduce the body's natural ability to fight off opportunistic intestinal pathogens by disrupting the normal bacterial layer's colonization resistance abilities. Stress can do this by increasing certain hormones in the body that regulate epithelial permeability (or how easily nutrients pass through the cell walls),[50] which, in turn, affects the composition of the normal flora in your intestines.[51-53]

Probiotics can reduce stress-related changes that occur in your body. Lactobacilli probiotics have been shown to correct structural changes in the cell surfaces of the intestines brought on by stress and restore the ability of bacterial adherence to intestinal walls, thus aiding the restoration of the bacterial barrier effect disrupted by stress factors.[54-56]

Recommendations for Stress

- Although evidence from animal models shows probiotics are effective in correcting some of the consequences of stress, human trials specifically studying probiotics and stress are needed.
- Indirect evidence from studies shows probiotics may be effective in treating conditions known to be triggered by stress (traveler's diarrhea, inflammatory bowel disease, and irritable bowel syndrome).

WEIGHT LOSS

Frequently Asked Questions

How can probiotics have an effect on weight loss?

Probiotics may be involved because of the benefit of calcium contained in yogurts.

Can probiotics help for weight loss?

No direct effect has been reported, but there may be some benefit if the probiotic is taken in a yogurt or other dairy product.

Probiotics have been proposed as aids to weight loss.[57] Some preliminary evidence has shown an association between calcium levels in the diet and weight loss.[58,59] A recent study showed more weight loss in a group that consumed yogurt compared to a group that consumed the same amount of calories and calcium (as tablets).[60] Probiotics ingested in yogurts may help with weight reduction, but it

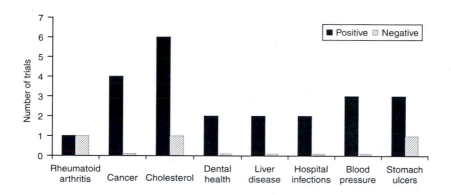

FIGURE 8.2. Summary of positive and negative randomized controlled trials testing probiotics for various diseases and conditions.

remains to be seen whether this is a direct effect of the probiotic or other substances in the yogurt.

Recommendations for Weight Loss

- Clinical trials are needed to see whether probiotics are helpful for weight loss.
- Daily consumption of a good nonfat, living-culture yogurt provides essential nutrients and may help in a weight-loss program that includes calorie reduction and exercise.

CONCLUSION

Probiotics are not "miracle drugs," and they do not work for all diseases. Probiotics show the most promise in reducing or eliminating diseases that result from some disturbance of normal microbial flora or involve the immune system. Evidence supports some health claims (see Figure 8.2), but others require more study. In addition, different probiotics need to be studied, as only a few strains have been targeted by researchers.

Chapter 9

Probiotic Products on the Market

This chapter provides examples of commercially available probiotic products in the United States and elsewhere, and the information useful in deciding which ones to buy. This listing is not all-inclusive since many probiotic products come on the market regularly, nor does inclusion on the list indicate or imply endorsement of any specific product by the authors.

In the past ten years, the number of commercially available probiotic products in the United States has tripled to more than 300. There are even more probiotic products available in other countries, especially in Europe and Asia. Some are available worldwide via the Internet, while others are available only in retail outlets (grocery stores, pharmacies, natural food stores, supplement stores, etc.). Examples of commercially available probiotic products are given, as well as some positive and cautionary points for each. The authors do not endorse specific products listed in this chapter; they are simply providing examples.

FREQUENTLY ASKED QUESTIONS

Are the probiotic products sold in the United States different from those sold in other countries?

They may appear to be different, but what appears on the product label varies from country to country, owing to regulatory differences. Most of the probiotic products on the market contain lactobacilli strains, a yeast, or mixtures of these.

The Power of Probiotics
© 2007 by The Haworth Press, Inc. All rights reserved.
doi:10.1300/5597_09

Can probiotics come in several forms?

Yes. Probiotics can be added to a food product or may be used in fermentation to make food. To be considered a probiotic product, living organisms must be present in the final food product and should provide some health benefit. Probiotics also may be sold in capsules of dried or freeze-dried (lyophilized) powder made from cultures grown in a laboratory. Probiotics may be sold as a single microorganism or as mixtures of several types of microorganisms.

What is the difference between dried and freeze-dried products?

Probiotic tablets or capsules are made from liquid cultures of microbes that are centrifuged (spun at high speeds) to harvest just the solids. The microbes can be simply dried by heat or air or can be lyophilized (vacuum-dried in the frozen state). Lyophilized products are stable over long periods of time, whereas air- or heat-dried products lose potency during processing.

Some probiotics list "FOS" on the label. What is this?

"FOS," or fructooligosaccharide, is a prebiotic. Prebiotics are used to help probiotic organisms grow in the body. Essentially, they are food for the probiotic microbes.

Are probiotics in food products better than those in capsules?

Not necessarily. Probiotics in food products usually require refrigeration and have shorter shelf lives (weeks to months) than capsules (one to two years). Also, probiotics in dairy products should not be taken by people who are lactose intolerant unless the probiotic produces lactase, which can break down lactose.

How does one find a good probiotic product?

This is discussed in Chapter 10. While probiotic products are widely available, finding a good product requires some research and study by the consumer.

ALPHABETICAL LISTING OF PROBIOTICS

The following are examples of commercially available probiotic products. This list is not all-inclusive, but provides a description of representative products (see Figure 9.1).

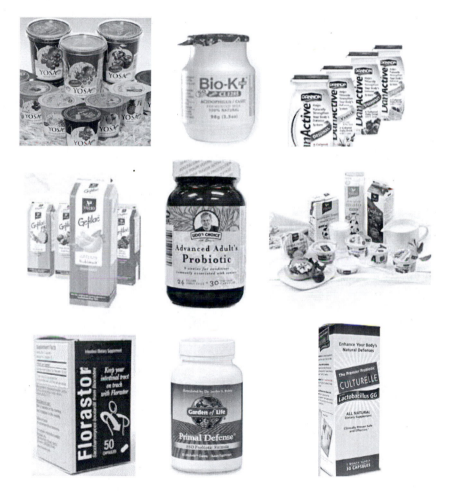

FIGURE 9.1. Examples of probiotic products. *Source:* Photograph by Lynne V. McFarland.

Acidophilus. These tablets are manufactured by Nature Made (Pharmavite), a U.S. company. These are *Lactobacillus acidophilus* tablets, each containing 500 million viable cells.
- A positive note: Pharmavite is a large, reputable company that participates in the U.S. Pharmacopeia dietary supplement program to assure product quality.

Acidophilus and Bifidus Adult Formula CR-1. These capsules are manufactured by Custom Probiotics, Glendale, California. Capsules contain *Lactobacillus acidophilus, L. plantarum, L. rhamnosus, Bifidobacterium bifidum,* and *B. longum* at a potency of at least 25 billion viable bacteria per capsule. No specific health claims are stated.
- A positive note: Potent probiotic mixture made by a reputable company.

Acidophilus Tykmaelk Fermented Milk. This milk product is manufactured by Klover, a Danish company. The milk is fermented with the probiotic *Lactobacillus acidophilus*. It is available in Europe, but not in the United States. See SWEET ACIDOPHILUS MILK.

Actilight. This product's health claim is to strengthen the body's natural defenses. It is available in many countries.
- A positive note: The manufacturer, Beghin-Say, is well established with years of experience and a varied product line.

Actimel. This is a yogurt manufactured by a French company, Danone, or the U.S.-based Dannon. The yogurt contains the probiotic *Lactobacillus acidophilus* (10^{10} live organisms per serving) and a prebiotic.

Activia. Flavored yogurts manufactured by Dannon, containing *Bifidobacterium animalis* (although the label calls this *"Bifidus regularis,"* which is not a scientifically approved name. Claims to "help slow intestinal transit." Available in the United States.

Align. Capsules of *Bifidobacterium infantis* 35624 are manufactured by Procter and Gamble. Function claim on the product is "to promote and maintain natural, healtlhy intestinal balance." Available in the United States over the Internet.

BifidoBiotics. This probiotic is manufactured by a U.S. Company—Allergy Research Group. Capsules contain *Lactobacillus sporogenes, L. rhamnosus, L. acidophilus, Bifidobacterium breve, B. longum,* and the prebiotic FOS. The potency is four billion organisms per capsule. It is available in the United States and via the Internet. No health claims are made for the product.

Bioflorin. This is manufactured by Sanofi Synthelabo. It contains *Enterococcus faecium SF68.* It is available in Europe.
- A positive note: This has been tested in clinical studies.

Bio-K+. This fermented milk product is manufactured by Bio-K+ International Inc., a Canadian company. The milk is sold in bottles of 100 g containing 50 million living bacteria (*Lactobacillus acidophilus* and *L. casei*). Its health claim is daily consumption "promotes and maintains a healthy and well-balanced digestive system."

Culturelle. This dietary supplement was distributed by ConAgra, a U.S. company, but sold to Amerifit Nutrition, Inc., in June 2006. Capsules contain lyophilized cultures of *Lactobacillus rhamnosus* strain GG (30 billion per capsule) and inulin, a plant-based prebiotic (oligosaccharide from chicory root). The manufacturer suggests taking this product "if you are under stress, taking antibiotics, traveling or simply want to promote your health." It is sold in the United States and via the Internet.
- Positive note: It was made by a large, well-established manufacturer (ConAgra) and uses a probiotic strain that has been subject to years of research and many clinical trials.

DanActive. These drinks are manufactured by Dannon, a U.S. company. These drinks contain the probiotic *Lactobacillus casei* (10^{10} live organisms per serving), *L. bulgaricus, L. casei,* and *Streptococcus thermophilus*. It is available in the United States and one of its health claims is to "naturally strengthen your body's defense system."
- Positive notes: The product has been used in several clinical trials with good results. It is made by respected manufacturer.
- A consideration: The product must be refrigerated.

EarthFlora. Manufactured by Life Science Products, Inc., a U.S. company, these capsules contain soil-based organisms (strains not given). Health claims include "stimulation of the immune system, reduces tissue damage in the heart, boosts nutritional assimilation, remission of numerous diseases including anemia, lung cancer, leukemia, lupus," etc. This product was relaunched with health claims that were better supported. Now it is sold as "Nature's Biotics."

- A cautionary note: Use caution when considering products with numerous health claims that are not supported by well-controlled scientific trials and go beyond regulations for dietary supplement health claims. Products with unsubstantiated claims are common on some Web sites.

***Enterococcus faecium* SF68.** See BIOFLORIN.

***Escherichia coli (E. coli)* Nissle 1917.** See MULTAFLOR.

Evolus. This fermented milk product is manufactured by Valio Ltd., a Finnish company. Milk is fermented with the probiotic strain *Lactobacillus rhamnosus* strain GG. Its health claim is "to control blood pressure." The product was launched in Iceland in 2000. It is not available in the United States.

- A positive note: It is made by respected manufacturer.
- A cautionary note: The probiotic strain used has been studied for other diseases, but there are few studies supporting a reduction in blood pressure.

Florastor. This dietary supplement is manufactured by Laboratoires Biocodex, a French company. Capsules contain lyophilized cultures of the probiotic *Saccharomyces boulardii*. It is available in 50-mg and 250-mg capsules. The 250-mg dose has been tested in numerous clinical trials. The product has a health claim that it "maintains balance of intestinal flora and promotes intestinal health." It is sold in the United States and via the Internet. It is sold throughout the world under numerous brand names. (Perenterol, Ultra-Levure, Bioflor, Floratil, etc.)

- Positive notes: Made by respected manufacturer with years of experience, it uses a probiotic strain of yeast that has been the subject of years of research and numerous clinical trials. It is sold by the manufacturer, who funded the original research.

Fungal Defense. Manufactured by Garden of Life, a U.S. company, this product is a mixture of "homeostatic soil organisms," various herbs (oregano, olive leaf extract, garlic, and yucca juice extracts) and minerals. The soil organisms are *Lactobacillus acidophilus, L. bulgaricus, L. lactis, L. plantarum, L. casei, Saccharomyces boulardii, Bifidobacterium bifidum, B. lichenformis,* and *Bacillus subtilus.* The health claim for this product is to "balance yeast overgrowth."

- Cautionary notes. Not all the organisms listed on the label are soil organisms. Not all the organisms listed on the label have been scientifically studied for *Candida* yeast infections. It has numerous nonprobiotic ingredients for no apparent reason.

Gaio Soya. This yogurt is manufactured by MD Foods, a Danish company. It contains the probiotic referred to as Causido culture (two strains of *Enterococcus faecium* and two strains of *Streptococcus thermophilus*). This product has been popular in Denmark since its introduction in 1993. It was withdrawn in the United Kingdom because of unsatisfactory sales coupled with adverse media coverage surrounding claims that it lowers cholesterol and "may help reduce the risk of heart disease." It is, however, available in Europe.

Gefilus. This line of food products (milk, yogurts, cheese, and infant formula) is manufactured by Valio Ltd., a Finnish company. The dairy products contain the probiotic *Lactobacillus rhamnosus* strain GG. It is available in Europe. Health claims include "protects against gastrointestinal infections and imbalances in the body." It was launched in Finland in 1990.

- Positive notes: It is made by a well-respected manufacturer who has funded most of the original research. The probiotic strain has been extensively studied in good clinical trials.

Jarro-Dophilus EPS. These are capsules containing four lactobacillus strains, four bifidobacteria strains, *Lactococcus brevi, Pediococcus acidilactici* R1001, and *Lactococcus diacetylactis* R0100. Manufactured by Jarrow Formulas, Los Angeles, USA. The potency is 4.4 billion organisms per enteric-coated capsule.

- Positive notes: This is a potent product in specially coated capsules that reduce destruction by stomach acid. It is made by a respected producer of dietary supplements.
- A cautionary note: The rationale for benefit to human health for inclusion of the *Pediococcus* and *Lactococcus* strains in this product is unclear.

Jour après Jour. This is a skim milk manufactured by Lactel, a French dairy company. It is enriched with the branded prebiotic Actilight, from a French company, Beghin-Say. It is aimed at "women wishing to maintain or improve their health status through daily consumption of this product." It is available in Europe.

- A cautionary note: There is limited scientific evidence to support its rather broad health claim.

Lactobacillus acidophilus. See ACIDOPHILUS. This is available in many products.

Lactobacillus casei **Shirota.** See YAKULT.

Lactobacillus reuteri. See PROBIOTICA.

Lactobacillus rhamnosus **strain GG.** See CULTURELLE and GEFILUS.

LC1 Go. This powder, sprinkled on top of cold food, is manufactured by the major multinational food company Nestle. It contains the probiotic *Lactobacillus johnsonii*. Widely available in France (launched in 1994), Germany (has 60 percent market share), Switzerland, and Italy, its health claim is it "enhances the body's immune system, helps digestion and fights undesirable bacteria." This product was withdrawn from France and the United Kingdom following poor market response. LC1 Go was launched in the United States in 2000 but was recently withdrawn. A competing product, Actimel (Dannon), has done well. It is available in the United States as DanActive (see earlier entry in this list).

Multaflor. This is manufactured by Ardeypharm Herdecke, a German company, and Emonta, an Austrian company. *Escherichia coli* Nissle 1917, the strain used in this product, initially was isolated from a soldier in World War I who, unlike his comrades, did not contract enterocolitis. Each capsule contains at least 2.5 billion viable bacteria. Available in Europe, it has indications for ulcerative colitis, irritable colon, and constipation.

- A positive note: It has been tested in clinical trials.

Nature's Biotics. This dietary supplement is manufactured by Life Science Products in Utah. The label states that each capsule contains soil-based organisms (*Lactobacillus acidophilus, Bifidobacterium* *bifidum, Bacillus licheniformis, Bacillus subtilis, Lactobacillus lactis,* and *Lactobacillus bulgaricus).* Health claims are the product will "contribute to good health, breaks down hydrocarbons, produces proteins that act as antigen, aggressive against pathological molds, yeasts, fungi and viruses, helps eliminate toxic wastes, defends against infection and provides Lactoferrin supplementation."

- A cautionary note: These broad health claims are not supported by randomized clinical trials.

PB8. This dietary supplement is manufactured by Nutrition Now Inc., a Canadian company. These capsules contain a mixture of pro biotics: four strains of *Lactobacillus,* two strains of *Bifidobacterium* and two strains of *Streptococcus.* The health claim is "to maintain a healthy balance of intestinal flora."

- A cautionary note: The manufacturer did not fund original research.

Primal Defense. This dietary supplement is manufactured by Garden of Life, a U.S. company. These capsules contain 14 "homeostatic soil organisms," including ten strains of lactobacilli, *Bifidobacteria bifidum, Bacillus subtilis, Bacillus licheniformis,* and *Saccharomyces boulardii.* The product claims the soil organisms "colonize in the gut, eat through putrefied materials and pathogenic organisms. This colonization also inhibits the growth of these offensive bacteria, parasites and viruses, activates B-lympocyte production and has unique immune stimulating effects."

- Cautionary notes: These broad health claims are not supported by randomized clinical trials. Not all the organisms listed are soil organisms. The manufacturer has not funded original research.

Probiotic Plus Oligofructose. The yogurt is manufactured by Bauer, a German company. It contains the probiotics *Lactobacillus acidophilus* and *L. bifidus* type LA7 and the prebiotic Raftilose (an oligofructose). It is available in Europe.

Probiotica. This is a chewable dietary supplement sold by McNeil Consumer Healthcare, a U.S. company, and licensed from BioGaia Biologics, a Swedish company. These lemon-flavored chewable tablets contain the probiotic *Lactobacillus reuteri* (100 million cells per tablet). The health claims include "promoting digestive health and maintaining a healthy balance of 'friendly' bacteria in the digestive tract." This product, introduced in December 2000, is available in the United States. It is sold under the brand name "Reuteri tablets" in Europe.

- Positive notes: The manufacturer is well known and has years of experience. The probiotic strain has been well studied.

ProViva Drink. Manufactured by Skanemejerier, a Swedish company, and Dairy UK Ltd., a UK company, the drink contains the probiotic *Lactobacillus plantarum* strain 299v. Available in Europe, the stated health claims are "to help maintain the digestive system's natural balance and maintains a healthy immune system."

Saccharomyces boulardii. See FLORASTOR.

Sweet Acidophilus Milk. Sold in the United States by Purity Dairies, this contains the probiotic *Lactobacillus acidophilus* (~500 million in an 8 oz glass). The stated health claims are "prevents indigestion, reduces intestinal gas and helps prevent diarrhea and constipation."

- A cautionary note: The health claim to "prevent diarrhea and constipation" is not allowed by U.S. law. There are scientific trials using *Lactobacillus acidophilus* to treat diarrhea, but the current Dietary Supplement Health Education Act does not allow a dietary supplement to claim to prevent or treat any disease.

Symbalance. Manufactured by Tonilait, a Swiss company, this yogurt contains the probiotics *Lactobacillus reuteri, L. acidophilus,* and *L. casei,* and a prebiotic (an inulin powder extracted from chicory roots, which is a mixture of oligosaccharides). Available in Europe, this product claims it "helps prevent digestion blocks due to the overgrowth of the yeast *Candida albicans* in the GI [gastrointestinal] tract."

- A cautionary note: This health claim is not supported by published randomized clinical trials.

Total Body Support. This supplement is manufactured by Pure Health Systems, a U.S. company. Each capsule contains a mixture of eight probiotics, including *Lactobacillus bulgaricus, L. acidophilus* strain DDS-1, *L. plantarium,* and *B. bifidum,* and a prebiotic, FOS.

Health claims for this product include replenishing the immune system. Manufacturer recommendation is for antibiotic therapy, poor diets, vaginal and urinary tract infections, chronic liver disease, constipation, acne, lactose intolerance, and emotional stress.

- A cautionary note: The health claims are not supported by published clinical studies.

Udo's Choice Probiotic Blends. There are six probiotic products sold under this brand name. Manufactured by Flora Inc., a Canadian company, these products are dried cultures in capsules and may contain *Lactobacillus acidophilus, L. casei, L. plantarum, L. rhamnosus, L. salivarius, Bifidobacterium bifidum, B. breve, B. infantis, B. longum,* and *Streptococcus thermophilus.* Health claims include "limits the action of invading microbes and disease-causing bacteria, breaks down lactose, contributes to the absorption of minerals, improves digestion of proteins, carbohydrates and fat, improves immunological and inflammatory responses and promotes regular bowel movements."

- A cautionary note: The health claim to "limit disease-causing bacteria" is not strictly allowed by U.S. law. However, this claim is in a very grey area of claims that are allowable. What should raise a red flag is that this specific product's claims are not supported by randomized clinical trials.

VSL#3. Manufactured by Nature's Pharmaceuticals, Inc., a U.S. company, this is a probiotic preparation of freeze-dried lactic acid bacteria (*Lactobacillus casei, L. plantarum, L. acidophilus, L. bulgaricus, Bifidobacterium longum, B. breve, B. infantis, and Streptococcus thermophilus*). Each packet contains a total of 450 billion bacteria. The claim is "to provide healthy bacteria for the gastrointestinal tract."

- A positive note: Several good clinical trials have been conducted using this mixture.

Yakult. A citrus-flavored beverage manufactured by Yakult Honsha, a Japanese company, Yakult Europe BV, a Dutch company, and Korea Yakult LTD, this contains the probiotic *Lactobacillus casei* subspecies Shirota (10^8 cfu/ml). Available in Japan, Korea, and Europe, it was launched in 1996 in the United Kingdom. The basic health claim is that daily consumption of this beverage "leads to a healthier intestine and therefore a healthier body."

- Positive notes: It is made by a reputable manufacturer. This strain of *Lactobacillus* has been well studied and tested in humans.

Yeast Defense. A dietary supplement manufactured by Nutrition Now Inc., a Canadian company, the capsules contain the probiotic *Lactobacillus acidophilus,* along with 17 strains of fungi. The health claim is that it will "help the body combat yeast overgrowth and maintain a healthy balance of intestinal flora."

- Cautionary notes: The manufacturer did not fund original research. The product was not tested in clinical trials.

Yosa-Oat-based Desserts. Manufactured by Bioferme Oy, a Finnish company, these products are made from oat bran fermented by the probiotics *Lactobacillus acidophilus* and *Bifidobacterium bifidum*. These are available in Europe. The health claims for these products are "to improve the well-being of the body, balance the stomach and increase the natural resistance of the intestines."

- A positive note: This is an interesting way to deliver probiotics, other than capsules or dairy products.

CONCLUSION

Although a multitude of probiotic products are available, not all are of the same quality or effectiveness. Buyers should look for established manufacturers, the type of information given on the product label, reasonable health claims, and evidence to support these claims. The information in this book should provide a valuable guide when choosing which probiotic to use, but is not to be interpreted as an end assessment of any particular product.

Chapter 10

Buying the Best Product

Buying a probiotic product takes a little more effort than the typical medication obtained from a pharmacist. When a prescription drug or over-the-counter drug is purchased in the United States, the Food and Drug Administration (FDA) and the product's manufacturer have determined that it is clinically effective for what it claims to treat or prevent and is reasonably safe to take. In contrast, dietary supplements, such as probiotics, are not subject to this high standard of guarantee. They may be of high quality—many are—but the regulations and requirements for drugs and dietary supplements differ. The consumer should be better informed about these types of supplements. The authors believe that after reading this book, the consumer will be better equipped to buy a product that is both effective and safe.

FREQUENTLY ASKED QUESTIONS

Which probiotics are best?

Different probiotics have different effects, so selections should be based on the condition to be treated.

The Power of Probiotics
© 2007 by The Haworth Press, Inc. All rights reserved.
doi:10.1300/5597_10

Is there a difference between the various brands of probiotics?

Yes. Some brands are made by reputable manufacturers with high standards for quality control, safety, and effectiveness; others are not.

Should one be suspicious if manufacturers quote self-funded research?

Advertising brochures quoting the manufacturer's own unpublished research should be read with a critical eye. However, if the manufacturer has funded original research done at an independent university, then the results can be better trusted. If the research has been published in a well-known, peer-reviewed scientific journal, then it has been carefully scrutinized by other scientists (peers) who do not have a financial incentive to give a biased report. These findings can be trusted.

Does more expensive mean "better"?

No. The effectiveness of a probiotic is not related to price.

Do probiotics lose potency over time?

Yes. Look for an expiration date on the bottle or box. Products that are lyophilized (freeze-dried) are more active and have longer shelf lives (one to two years) than products that are air- or heat-dried.

Are the probiotics sold in capsules better than those sold as enriched foods?

Not necessarily. As shown in the previous chapter, probiotics are sold in a variety of delivery mechanisms: tablets, capsules, dairy products, lemon-flavored products, oatcakes, etc.

THE FIVE QUESTIONS

Choosing the right probiotic for you can be challenging, as illustrated in Figure 10.1. Because federal regulations do not require the

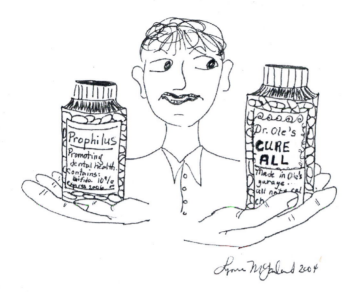

FIGURE 10.1. Choosing the right probiotic can be difficult. The Five Questions should be addressed. *Source:* Illustration by Lynne V. McFarland.

same strict testing standards for dietary supplements as for prescription and over-the-counter medications, there are fewer guarantees that the product on the shelf is safe or effective for the disease it claims to treat or prevent. So, the buyer should be prepared. There are five questions to be considered before choosing a probiotic, which are discussed in the following sections.

What is the indication or intended use for the probiotic?

In the United States, it is important to remember that probiotics are regulated as "dietary supplements" and, by law, cannot claim to "treat or prevent" a disease. They are allowed to state "structure or function claims" that allude to health benefits. For intestinal health, these claims commonly are "to promote intestinal health," "to regulate intestinal microflora," and "to insure intestinal balance." For skin diseases, allowable claims would say "promoting a healthy skin" or something similar. Probiotics cannot state specifically that they are effective, for example, for traveler's diarrhea, colitis, or antibiotic-associated diseases, even though there are good scientific studies that show some can effectively treat or prevent these diseases. It is more a business decision to sell probiotics as dietary supplements, as this saves the manufacturer the millions of dollars it costs to satisfy FDA requirements for new drugs. In other countries, more specific health claims may be permitted. Because of their broad biological activities, some probiotics may be effective for more than one disease.

The Five Questions:

1. *Indication?*
2. *Source?*
3. *Manufacturer?*
4. *Label?*
5. *Evidence?*

What is the source of the probiotic?

Where does one go to purchase an appropriate probiotic product? Retailers of probiotics can vary from the local supermarket to pharmacies to specialty natural food stores to the Internet. It is important to choose wisely where to purchase the product, as some vendors do not screen what they sell as carefully as others. Some retailers have committees to review each product for safety and possible liability issues before they put the products on their shelves, while others do not screen products as closely. Extra caution is needed for purchase of probiotics on the Internet because not all Web sites are connected to reputable sellers.

Who are the manufacturers of the probiotic?

Unlike FDA-approved prescription drugs and over-the-counter medications, there are few regulations for manufacturers of probiotics other than that the product not be adulterated (that is, no substances can be included that are not listed on the label) and the manufacturer meets food (not drug) good manufacturing practices. Some probiotics are made by companies that have businesslike names but no real experience making safe and reliable probiotic products. The best strategy is to choose a manufacturer that financed scientific studies published in reliable medical journals and is experienced in producing safe and consistent products. The manufacturer or company that funds reliable clinical trials can be found by looking at the original published studies. The manufacturer or supplier usually is listed in the part of the research paper titled "Methods," under the section describing the probiotic treatment, or listed in a footnote as a funding source. If a probiotic stated in the study is not available, a probiotic made by a company that has experience with other related products and is trusted should selected. Also, check with the Better Business Bureau in the United States to see whether the company has been the target of complaints. It is generally better to purchase probiotics of recognizable brand names rather than unknown generic products. Major manufacturers have vested interests in protecting their reputations and are less likely to compromise the quality of their probiotic product by using shortcut methods.

What type of information should the label contain?

A complete label is a good sign that the manufacturer has experience and knows how to produce a reliable product. In the United States, a probiotic label should have a reasonable structure or function claim. Probiotics can make either "body function claims," which are statements that relate to a normal bodily function, such as "helps to maintain good digestion," or "body structure claims," which relate to a body structure, such as "helps to promote bone health." Appropriate probiotic health claims can include "improves intestinal functioning," "enhances immune function," "improves skin health," or "replaces intestinal flora." Inappropriate claims such as "prevents cancer," "treats diarrhea," or "cures arthritis" should be a red flag indicating that the manufacturer is not complying with the law and this product should not be purchased. Inappropriate health claims can be due to overzealous marketing, ignorance of the law, or outright fraud.

The product label also should list the strains of the probiotics contained. A suspicious label is one that merely states "contains friendly bacteria" says nothing specifically about what types of probiotic strains are included. Look for specific names of bacteria, such as "contains *Lactobacillus rhamnosus*." Also, the label should state the potency of the probiotic, or the number of living microorganisms contained in a specific amount of product. The label might say: "Each capsule contains 2×10^{10} live *Saccharomyces boulardii*." This means that each capsule contains 20 billion viable yeast cells of *Saccharomyces boulardii*. Generally, choose a product that has 1 billion or more viable microbial cells per dose. The daily dose should be stated on the label, such as, "Take two capsules twice a day." Look for an expiration date on the label or bottle. Most probiotics are living organisms that are freeze-dried to extend their shelf lives. They can last for one to two years at room temperature. But the expiration date should always be given. A lot number should be on the bottle or box showing that the manufacturer can trace batches of probiotics to the source. This is needed if quality control issues arise should an investigation be called after the product is on the market. The manufacturer of the product and its location should be on the label. A good label provides enough information to know what the probiotic is good for, who makes it, how it should be taken, and whom to contact if questions arise. A label that does not have this information should arouse suspicion.

Some stores carry printed information and handouts about the dietary supplements they sell. Be careful in determining whether the literature cites valid scientific data for its claims or is merely a sales pitch with no verifiable research to support it. The same scrutiny must be applied to probiotics sold on the Internet.

What type of evidence supports the probiotic product?

The greatest confidence in safety and effectiveness lies with those probiotics that are subject to sound scientific studies, the results of which are published in peer-reviewed scientific journals (or this book!). Probiotics that contain strains of bacteria or yeast that have not been studied in humans offer no evidence of their effectiveness or safety. Be suspicious of probiotics with health claims that are not supported by good scientific studies. Probiotics that have been subject to scientific scrutiny are described in this book.

WHERE TO FIND INFORMATION

In addition to this book, there are several good sources of information about probiotics. Libraries can provide both texts and research papers concerning probiotics and scientific studies related to them. The Internet also can be a good gateway to information. The following Web addresses may be useful:

www.fda.gov—This is the Web site of the U.S. FDA. It provides a wide array of information pertaining to research, studies, findings, and reviews relating to the FDA.

http://ods.od.nih.gov—This is the Web site of the National Institutes of Health, providing information on health resources, clinical trials, drug information, and a large list of other health- and research-related topics. Look under "Office of Dietary Supplements" for information on probiotics.

www.ncbi.nlm.nih.gov/entrez, or PubMed—This is a Web site operated by the National Library of Medicine. PubMed contains a database of biomedical articles. Enter "probiotic" and the name of the medical condition in the search box.

health.nih.gov—Enter the National Institutes of Health Web site and search under "Alternative Medicine" or "National Center for Complementary and Alternative Medicine." There is a wealth of material on dietary supplements, probiotics, and other types of natural medicines.

USprobiotics.org—This is a resource site for activities, research, and developments in probiotics and dairy products, which is written by an authority on probiotics and is nicely organized.

Consumerlab.com—This Web site provides results of laboratory testing of consumer products including probiotics in order to assess product quality. This is a subscription service site, but some useful information on product quality is available at no charge. This is a very useful resource for the consumer wishing to select a quality product. Unfortunately, only a limited number of probiotics have been selected for testing.

Alternatively, using the search engine of your choice, type in "probiotics," "probiotics+research," "probiotics+information," "probiotics+(name of disease)," or something similar, and check what is available.

CONCLUSION

With a little preparation, the right probiotic can be chosen with confidence. Researching and getting the right kinds of information improve the likelihood of selecting a good product and having positive outcome with its use.

Chapter 11

Safety of Probiotics

There are risks in consuming living microorganisms for therapeutic purposes; however, the risks are small. Billions of microbes in food and water are swallowed every day, usually without harm. Risks from probiotics are rare, but may be present if a contaminant enters during manufacturing and packaging or if the user has a severely weakened immune system. In most cases, probiotics can be used with little concern regarding risk.

FREQUENTLY ASKED QUESTIONS

If a probiotic containing billions of living microorganisms is consumed, what is the risk for overgrowth and infection?

Most probiotic strains do not persist in the intestines for longer than two to three weeks. Much of the ingested dose is killed during the passage through the intestinal tract. Usually, enough probiotic microorganisms are left alive to be effective, but not enough to be harmful.

Can one easily overdose on a probiotic?

An overdose would be difficult with commercially available products. Only so many living microbes can be packed into a capsule or

The Power of Probiotics
© 2007 by The Haworth Press, Inc. All rights reserved.
doi:10.1300/5597_11

tablet. The body can easily handle three or four doses of a good probiotic on a daily basis with no ill effects.

How does one choose a safe probiotic?

Brand familiarity, as with other products, is important. Brands that are backed by good scientific studies can be trusted over brands that have not been subject to human studies. Product selection is discussed in Chapter 10.

Are probiotics safe for children?

Generally, yes. Studies support general safety in use by children. In rare cases, children who were extremely ill have been reported to have had problems with probiotic products.

Are probiotics safe for adults?

Generally, yes. Studies support the general safety of probiotics for use by adults. People ranging from healthy volunteers to extremely ill elderly patients have taken probiotics with few significant adverse effects.

Are probiotics safe for pets?

Yes, probiotics have been successfully given to a wide variety of animals (cats, cows, dogs, horses, bear, chicken, and rodents).

Are probiotics beneficial to pets?

Much of the early research on probiotics involved animals. Probiotics are being studied by the U.S. Department of Agriculture to improve the health of some newborn animals.

RISKS IN GENERAL

Safety information can be gathered from several sources. One can find some safety information on the label of a product (see Figure 11.1)

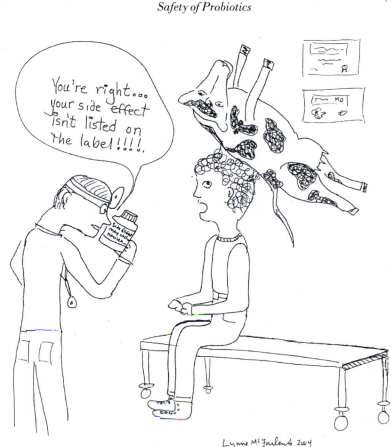

FIGURE 11.1. Not all effects may be listed on the product label. *Source:* Illustration by Lynne V. McFarland.

or in the package insert (an included paper that describes how to use the product and includes any safety concerns). In addition, a search of the medical literature may yield reports of risks or safety problems. In some cases, the U.S. government (usually the Food and Drug Administration [FDA]) may have information on the safety of the product. In the United States, probiotics added to foods are considered food additives with "Generally Recognized As Safe," or GRAS, status. This does not mean that all probiotics are considered GRAS—it refers to only those probiotics that are added to foods. This includes safe lactic-acid-producing bacteria, such as *Lactobacillus acidophilus, L. bulgaricus, L. fermentus, L. lactis,* and *Streptococcus thermophilus,* used in yogurts and buttermilks. *Lactobacillus rhamnosus* GG and bifidobacteria are not on this food additive list but have been well tested. Probiotics sold in capsules or tablets are considered "dietary supplements" in the United States and not considered GRAS, as they are not added to foods. For dietary supplements, it not required to provide extensive proof of safety and efficacy. It is the burden of government regulatory authorities to show that a probiotic product is not safe. As discussed in Chapter 1, the strict regulations for safety and efficacy mandated by the FDA for prescription and over-the-counter medications are not required for probiotics sold as dietary supplements.

When considering the "safety" of probiotics, several factors should be taken into account: The probiotic's ability to cause disease (pathogenicity), to produce damaging substances (virulence factors such as toxins), and to produce metabolic activities that might interfere with the body's normal functioning, and problems with quality control should also be considered. Most nonprobiotic drugs (such as prescription medications and over-the-counter drugs) cause some adverse effects, some quite serious, but the drug is used anyway because its therapeutic benefit is judged to be greater than the risk from side effects. This same sort of balanced judgment should used when considering the safety of probiotics.

Potential risks of probiotics:

- *Contamination*
- *Poor potency*
- *Unproven claims*
- *No strong federal oversight*
- *Adverse effects*
- *Infection*

Probiotic preparations have been used for many decades in Europe and Asia, where people are quite used to taking them for many reasons. Researching the reported literature for this book revealed that, in Europe and Asia, over 200 billion doses of probiotic doses have been purchased, yet fewer than 30 cases of serious adverse effects were reported. This is a remarkably good safety record. In the United

States, probiotics are relatively new on the market, but many have been studied in controlled clinical trials. In addition, studies in animals have looked at how probiotics interact with normal microbial flora in the intestine, vagina, and mouth, and on the skin. Commonly used probiotics have not been associated with excessive damage to tissues or disruption of beneficial normal microbial flora. Extensive testing has shown probiotics are well tolerated by animals, both healthy and those compromised by illness or stress. Nearly all probiotic products used in clinical trials also have been subject to extensive in vitro (laboratory) research and testing in animal models. These tests showed that the probiotics studied were neither pathogenic nor invasive, did not produce substances that can cause disease (such as toxins), and did not interfere with normal metabolic functioning.[1-4]

REPORTED ADVERSE EFFECTS

From Clinical Studies

The safety of most probiotics has been extensively reviewed. The general conclusion is that pathogenic potential is low and probiotics are generally safe to use. The advantage of years of careful research is that, although safety studies are not required, subjects who participate in clinical studies were carefully followed up for any adverse reactions. The large clinical studies have not reported serious problems with the probiotics that were given. For example, in one clinical study of 124 patients treated with *S. boulardii* (1 g/day for 28 days), five reported increased thirst (9 percent) and eight reported constipation (14 percent), whereas there were no reports of increased thirst and there were two of constipation in the placebo group. No other adverse effects were reported by either group.[5]

From Case Reports

There are isolated case reports of adverse effects associated with probiotic use.[4] These are discussed in the following text by the type of probiotic, and summarized in Table 11.1. A case report of adverse effects usually is a brief description of one or two patients who have developed an unusual illness or a rare side effect. However, these

TABLE 11.1. Reported types of adverse effects of probiotics from medical literature.

Probiotic product	Number of cases	Type of side effect and underlying health status	Strain causing disease identified as same strain as probiotic	Reference
Probiotic yogurt (supermarket brand, daily serving not given nor type of probiotic identified)	1	Fatal septicemia in 42-year-old woman immunocompromised, with recurrent *Clostridium difficile* disease and renal failure	*Lactobacillus rhamnosus* identified in blood infection	Note 6
Lactobacillus rhamnosus GG in probiotic dairy drink (1/2 liter per day, taken for 4 months)	1	Liver abscess in 74-year-old woman with multiple medical conditions. Recovered with antibiotic treatment	*Lactobacillus rhamnosus* GG in milk and strain causing liver abscess, identified as the same	Note 7
Lactobacillus probiotic	2	*Lactobacillus* bacteremia in two children with short gut syndrome taking probiotic. Recovered with antibiotics	*Lactobacillus* in blood and probiotic not identified	Note 8
Saccharomyces boulardii probiotic capsules (doses varied from 500 to 2000 mg/day)	14 from 1991-2000	Fungemia (fever and yeast in the blood) in all. All patients had been hospitalized with multiple conditions and central venous catheter	Only six had positive identification as *S. boulardii* in blood	Note 9

brief descriptions are not scientific proof that the adverse effect is due to the probiotic.

Bacillus *Probiotics*

One report documented three patients at a hospital in Germany who experienced diarrhea after taking a probiotic product containing *Bacillus cereus*.[10] However, investigators discovered two of the patients had diarrhea before they took the probiotic, so even though the bacillus strain isolated from the stools was identified as the same bacillus strain in the probiotic, it is unlikely that the probiotic strain caused diarrhea in two of the three cases. This illustrates the difficulty of assigning the cause of an illness when the same probiotic strain is found naturally in the body or in the environment.

Bifidobacterium Probiotics

No adverse effects from bifidobacterial probiotic products have been reported to date.

Enterococcal Probiotics

There have been no reports of risks from probiotics products containing enterococci, but there is some concern about routine use of enterococcal probiotics. This is because other enterococci strains of bacteria have caused bloodborne infections (septicemia), endocarditis (infection of the heart lining), and wound infections. However, the probiotic enterococci have not been associated with any of these serious infections. Another issue with routine enterococci probiotic use is the potential for spread of antibiotic-resistant strains of bacteria. In the United States, vancomycin-resistant enterococci are the most common cause of hospital-acquired infections. Enterococci, in general, are highly resistant to many antibiotics, but there is no current evidence to show that the enterococcal strains causing hospital infections are the same as those found in probiotics. However, if an infection with probiotic enterococci were to occur, it would be difficult to treat. Only careful surveillance may detect a problem. Another concern is the ability of enterococci to donate to other intestinal bacteria the genes that code for antibiotic resistance. This could lead to the spread of antibiotic resistance if the use of enterococcal probiotics becomes common, but there is no direct evidence for this. Enterococcal-based probiotics are not commercially available in the United States.

Lactobacillus *Probiotics*

Lactobacilli bacteria are present in many foods and part of our normal microflora. Lactobacilli strains used in probiotic products have an excellent safety record. Other lactobacilli strains, not used as probiotics, have been occasionally linked to human disease (usually endocarditis) in patients with compromised health. In 1990, *Lacto-*

bacillus rhamnosus GG became widely available in Finland as a probiotic product. Surveys for infections were conducted to address possible safety concerns stemming from widespread use of this probiotic. One researcher who reviewed all 3,317 cases of bacteria-positive blood cultures in Finland from 1989 to 1992 found only eight cases of bacteremia caused by lactobacilli bacteria. However, none of these were the types of strains used in Finnish probiotics.[11] A more recent look at the bacteremia cases in Finland, from 1995 to 2000, found only 11 cases of *Lactobacillus-rhamnosus*-GG-associated bacteremia cases, an annual incidence of 0.05/100,000/year.[12] Patients who developed *Lactobacillus* GG bacteremia were more likely to have severe or fatal comorbidities or surgeries or were immunosuppressed.[13] Other than the blood, lactobacilli probiotics have been isolated in only one other unexpected body site. To date, there has been one case reported of a person taking *Lactobacillus rhamnosus* GG who developed a liver abscess caused by this strain of probiotic.[7] Over the years, lactobacilli probiotics have been given to a variety of study populations, such as children, enteral (tube-fed) premature infants, elderly patients, patients with AIDS, hospitalized patients with multiple conditions, and otherwise healthy individuals, such as travelers and nonhospitalized adults, with only rare adverse effects reported.[4]

Saccharomyces *Probiotics*

This probiotic has been used in Europe for over 50 years. Reports of adverse effects are rare. *Saccharomyces boulardii* has been associated with rare cases of fungemia (fever and the presence of yeast in the bloodstream). All patients who developed fungemia had been hospitalized with multiple conditions and illnesses, and often had a history of surgery or broad-spectrum antibiotic use.[4,9] Of the 14 cases reported over the past 25 years, 3 were children under the age of two years and 11 were adults. All 14 were ill enough to require central venous catheters to deliver antibiotics or nutritional liquids directly into the bloodstream. All recovered from the fungemia, either by taking an antifungal medication or stopping the probiotic. A researcher investigating these cases of *S. boulardii* fungemia found that the yeast gained entry into the blood not by traveling out of the intestine and invading the rest of the body, but through contamination of the central catheter.[9] The probiotic was given to hospitalized patients who could not drink or eat by opening the probiotic capsules at their bedside and mixing it with their enteral tube solution. As these microorganisms are easily airborne, opening the capsules at bedside could have contaminated a wound or catheter site. As this is a potential problem, capsules for patients with catheters or open wounds should be opened and mixed in a different room. No other serious adverse effects have been reported for *S. boulardii*.

QUALITY CONTROL

The U.S. government does not require proof of strain identification, sterility, stability, and general safety for probiotics before they are sold as dietary supplements. This lack of tight regulation has led to quality control problems with some probiotics sold in the United States. Several studies have documented that the probiotic strains listed on the label may not actually be contained in the product.[14] In one study, at least one contaminant was present in 11 of 16 probiotics tested, and only 4 of the 16 had the correct lactobacillus strain claimed on the label.[15] In another case, we tested a probiotic product that claimed to contain "a multitude of probiotic strains," but upon testing the capsules were found to contain only sterile soil.

Confidence about the presence of the correct probiotic strain in the product is important for several reasons:

- Similar but different strains of microbes are known to cause disease.
- Only some strains have beneficial effects against disease.
- Waste of economic resources if not effective.

Some nonprobiotic strains of lactobacillus, enterococcus, and saccharomyces have been, on rare occassions, linked to disease. Proper microbiologic identification is necessary to guarantee that the strain listed on the probiotic label is not one of the disease-causing strains. The therapeutic effect of probiotics strains usually is not shared by strains that are otherwise closely related. In addition, if the product is not effective, time and money are wasted before effective treatment

can be started. Unfortunately, finding the incorrect strain in a probiotic product is not as uncommon as one might hope (see Table
11.2). As probiotics are a preparation of living organisms, batches of
organisms grow better at some times than others. This leads to
"batch-to-batch" variation, and may result in probiotic batches that
are not effective in preventing disease or have a lower potency than

TABLE 11.2. Examples of quality control problems in commercial probiotic
products.

Type of probiotic product	Probiotic claimed on the label	Problem in quality control	Reference
Lactinex	*L. acidophilus* and *L. bulgaricus*	Some batches of probiotic had no therapeutic effect	Note 16
Biosubtyl	*Bacillus subtilis*	Strain was different than labeled	Note 17
Enterogermina	*Bacillus subtilis*	Strain was different than labeled	Note 17
Not given	*Lactobacillus acidophilus*	No live organisms	Note 18
Review of 13 probiotic products sold in Britain	Various probiotic strains	Only 15% correctly labeled, 85% had bacteria not on label, lacked the labeled strain, only one-tenth the dose on label, or were below stated potency	Note 18
Review of 52 probiotic products in Britain	Various probiotic strains	Had bacteria not on label, lacked the labeled strain, and had less than the stated potency	Note 19
16 probiotics products in US for "restoring vaginal flora"	*Lactobacillus acidophilus*	75% labeled with wrong strain, 69% had at least one contaminant	Note 15
26 yogurts and probiotic diary products in Germany	Various *Lactobacillus* strains	Viable (living) dose varied from label, Lactobacilli strains other than labeled	Note 20
29 probiotic products	Various *Lactobacillus* strains	48% strains different than labeled	Note 21
9 health food products from United States or Canada	Various *Lactobacillus* strains	One-third had strain different than the labeled, and one-third had contaminants	Note 22

what is claimed on the label. A certain amount of latitude is allowed because the usual dose is billions of organisms per day. But when the result is a loss of effectiveness to prevent or treat disease, this can have a great impact. It is up to the probiotic manufacturers to "police" their own quality control and try to ensure that their product is all they claim it to be. Unfortunately, not all manufacturers have high-quality standards.

Generally, probiotics that have been extensively studied with controlled clinical trials at accredited medical centers have the best records of good quality control and reliability. Clinical trials are expensive, and the researchers and agencies funding the studies must be guaranteed the researched strain is the same strain of probiotic used in future products. Quality control for probiotics used in clinical trials, therefore, is usually higher. Also, probiotics that consist of a single strain have a more reliable record than mixtures of different strains of probiotics.[23]

CONTRAINDICATIONS

Consumers allergic to yeast should not use probiotics that contain yeast strains. These will have *"Saccharomyces"* listed as an ingredient on the label. Consumers intolerant of lactose (milk sugar) should not use probiotics that are sold in dairy products, such as milk beverages or yogurts.

SPECIAL CONCERNS

Although use during pregnancy or while nursing has not been specifically studied, probiotics have been widely used by pregnant and nursing women with no apparent ill effects. Use of probiotics by extremely ill patients, patients with impaired immune systems, and hospitalized children should be carefully supervised. The risks are low, but there have been rare cases of bacteremia or fungemia in these populations.

DRUG INTERACTIONS

If one is taking an antimicrobial, the antibiotic might inhibit or kill the probiotic microbe being used. Antibiotics are likely to kill or inhibit bacterial probiotics such as those containing lactobacilli, bifidobacteria, or streptococci. Antifungal drugs such as fluconazole or terbinafine can kill yeast probiotics such as those containing *Saccharomyces* species. A physician or pharmacist should be consulted to determine the likelihood of an antimicrobial interaction with a specific probiotic. One advantage of a yeast probiotic is that yeast will not be affected by an antibiotic. Antifungals will affect yeast, but antifungal therapy is less common than antibiotic therapy. The timing of the probiotic dose can help lessen these types of interactions. A probiotic taken at least two to three hours before or after an antibiotic or antifungal would decrease direct exposure of the probiotic to the antimicrobial.

CONCLUSIONS AND OBSERVATIONS

Probiotics generally are extremely safe, as evidenced by extensive research and a long history of safe use by a wide variety of people of all ages. Most concerns with probiotic safety can be minimized with selection of effective probiotic products using high-quality-control standards to ensure a pure, potent product. Adverse effects, though rare, justify continued surveillance of probiotics, especially as newer probiotics are introduced to the market.

Notes

Chapter 1

1. Metchnikoff E. *Prolongation of Life: Optimistic Studies*. Putnam and Sons, 1908.

2. Reid G, Sanders ME, Gaskins HR, Gibson GR, Mercenier A, Rastall R, Roberfroid M, Rowland I, Cherbut C, Klaenhammer TR. New scientific paradigms for probiotics and prebiotics. *Journal of Clinical Gastroenterology* 2003;37: 105-118.

3. McFarland LV. Normal flora: Diversity and functions. *Microbial Ecology in Health and Disease* 2000;12:193-207.

4. Elmer GW, Surawicz CM, McFarland LV. Biotherapeutic agents. A neglected modality for the treatment and prevention of selected intestinal and vaginal infections. *Journal of American Medical Association* 1996;275:870-876.

5. Dunne C, O'Mahony L, Murphy L, Thornton G, Morrissey D, O'Halloran S, Feeney M, Flynn S, Fitzgerald G, Daly C, et al. In vitro selection criteria for probiotic bacteria of human origin: Correlation with in vivo findings. *American Journal of Clinical Nutrition* 2001;73:386S-392S.

6. McFarland LV. Quality Control and Regulatory Issues for Biotherapeutic Agents. In: Elmer GW, McFarland LV, Surawicz CM, eds. *Biotherapeutic Agents and Infectious Diseases*. Totowa, NJ: Humana Press, 1999:1-26.

7. Silva M, Jacobus NV, Deneke C, Gorbach SL. Antimicrobial substance from a human Lactobacillus strain. *Antimicrobial Agents and Chemotherapy* 1987;31: 1231-1233.

8. Goldin BR, Gorbach SL, Saxelin M, Barakat S, Gualtieri L, Salminen S. Survival of Lactobacillus species (strain GG) in human gastrointestinal tract. *Digestive Diseases and Sciences* 1992;37:121-128.

9. Alander M, Satokari R, Korpela R, Saxelin M, Vilpponen-Salmela T, Mattila-Sandholm T, von Wright A. Persistence of colonization of human colonic mucosa by a probiotic strain, *Lactobacillus rhamnosus* GG, after oral consumption. *Applied and Environmental Microbiology* 1999;65:351-354.

10. Meurman JH, Antila H, Korhonen A, Salminen S. Effect of *Lactobacillus rhamnosus* strain GG (ATCC-53103) on the growth of *Streptococcus sobrinus* in vitro. *European Journal of Oral Sciences* 1995;103:253-258.

11. Meurman JH, Antila H, Salminen S. Recovery of Lactobacillus strain-GG (ATCC-53103) from saliva of healthy-volunteers after consumption of yogurt prepared with the bacterium. *Microbial Ecology in Health and Disease* 1994;7:295-298.

12. Wolf BW, Garleb KA, Ataya DG, Casas IA. Safety and tolerance of *Lactobacillus reuteri* in healthy adult male subjects. *Microbial Ecology in Health and Disease* 1995;8:41-50.

13. Casas I, Dobrogosz W. Validation of the probiotic concept: *Lactobacillus reuteri* confers broad-spectrum protection against disease in humans and animals. *Microbial Ecology in Health and Disease* 2000;12:247-285.

14. Sui J, Leighton S, Busta F, Brady L. 16S ribosomal DNA analysis of the faecal lactobacilli composition of human subjects consuming a probiotic strain *Lactobacillus acidophilus* NCFM (R). *Journal of Applied Microbiology* 2002; 93:907-912.

15. Asahara T, Nomoto K, Watanuki M, Yokokura T. Antimicrobial activity of intraurethrally administered probiotic *Lactobacillus casei* in a murine model of *Escherichia coli* urinary tract infection. *Antimicrobial Agents and Chemotherapy* 2001;45:1751-1760.

16. de Waard R, Garssen J, Bokken GCAM, Vos JG. Antagonistic activity of *Lactobacillus casei* strain Shirota against gastrointestinal *Listeria monocytogenes* infection in rats. *International Journal of Food Microbiology* 2002;73:93-100.

17. Hori T, Kiyoshima J, Shida K, Yasui H. Augmentation of cellular immunity and reduction of influenza virus titer in aged mice fed *Lactobacillus casei* strain Shirota. *Clinical and Diagnostic Laboratory Immunology* 2002;9:105-108.

18. Park MJ, Kim JS, Jung HC, Song IS, Lee JJ. The suppresive effect of a fermented milk containing lactobacilli on *Helicobacter pylori* in human gastric mucosa. *Gastroenterology* 2001;120:A590.

19. Spanhaak S, Havenaar R, Schaafsma G. The effect of consumption of milk fermented by *Lactobacillus casei* strain Shirota on the intestinal microflora and immune parameters in humans. *European Journal of Clinical Nutrition* 1998;52: 899-907.

20. Shimakawa Y, Matsubara S, Yuki N, Ikeda M, Ishikawa F. Evaluation of *Bifidobacterium breve* strain Yakult-fermented soymilk as a probiotic food. *International Journal of Food Microbiology* 2003;81:131-136.

21. Lund B, Edlund C, Barkholt L, Nord CE, Tvede M, Poulsen RL. Impact on human intestinal microflora of an *Enterococcus faecium* probiotic and vancomycin. *Scandinavian Journal of Infectious Diseases* 2000;32:627-632.

22. McFarland LV, Bernasconi P. *Saccharomyces boulardii*—A review of an innovative biotherapeutic agent. *Microbial Ecology in Health and Disease* 1993;6: 157-171.

23. Blehaut H, Massot J, Elmer GW, Levy RH. Disposition kinetics of *Saccharomyces boulardii* in man and rat. *Biopharmaceutics & Drug Disposition* 1989;10: 353-364.

24. Elmer GW, Moyer KA, Vega R, Surawicz CM, Collier AC, Hooton TM, McFarland LV. Evaluation of *Saccharomyces boulardii* for patients with HIV-related chronic diarrhea and in healthy volunteers receiving antifungals. *Microecology and Therapy* 1995;25:157-171.

25. Castagliuolo I, Riegler MF, Valenick L, Lamont JT, Pothoulakis C. *Saccharomyces boulardii* protease inhibits the effects of *Clostridium difficile* toxins A and B in human colonic mucosa. *Infection and Immunity* 1999;67:302-307.

26. Qamar A, Aboudola S, Warny M, Michetti P, Pothoulakis C, Lamont JT, Kelly CP. *Saccharomyces boulardii* stimulates intestinal immunoglobulin A immune response to *Clostridium difficile* toxin A in mice. *Infection and Immunity* 2001;69:2762-2765.

27. Buts JP, Bernasconi P, Vancraynest MP, Maldague P, Demeyer R. Response of human and rat small intestinal-mucosa to oral-administration of *Saccharomyces boulardii*. *Pediatric Research* 1986;20:192-196.

28. McFarland LV. A review of the evidence of health claims for biotherapeutic agents. *Microbial Ecology in Health and Disease* 2000;12:65-76.

Chapter 2

1. Cheng AC, Thielman NM. Update on traveler's diarrhea. *Current Infectious Disease Reports* 2002;4:70-77.

2. Rendi-Wagner P, Kollaritsch H. Drug prophylaxis for travelers' diarrhea. *Clinical Infectious Diseases* 2002;34:628-633.

3. Cavalcanti A, Clemens SA, Von Sonnenburg F, Collard F, De Clercq N, Steffen R, Clemens R. Traveler's diarrhea: Epidemiology and impact on visitors to Fortaleza, Brazil. *Revista Panamericana de Salud Pública* 2002;11:245-252.

4. Ilnyckyj A, Balachandra B, Elliott L, Choudhri S, Duerksen DR. Post-traveler's diarrhea irritable bowel syndrome: A prospective study. *American Journal of Gastroenterology* 2003;98:596-599.

5. Hill DR. Occurrence and self-treatment of diarrhea in a large cohort of Americans traveling to developing countries. *American Journal of Tropical Medicine and Hygiene* 2000;62:585-589.

6. Centers for Disease Control and Prevention (CDC) Health Information for International Travel, 2003-2004. Atlanta, Georgia: US Department of Health and Human Services, Public Health Services, 2004.

7. Adachi JA, Mathewson JJ, Jiang ZD, Ericsson CD, DuPont HL. Enteric pathogens in Mexican sauces of popular restaurants in Guadalajara, Mexico, and Houston, Texas. *Annals of Internal Medicine* 2002;136:884-887.

8. DuPont HL, Jiang ZD, Ericsson CD, Adachi JA, Mathewson JJ, DuPont MW, Palazzini E, Riopel LM, Ashley D, Martinez-Sandoval F. Rifaximin versus ciprofloxacin for the treatment of traveler's diarrhea: A randomized, double-blind clinical trial. *Clinical Infectious Diseases* 2001;33:1807-1815.

9. Guerrant RL, Steiner TS, Lima AA, Bobak DA. How intestinal bacteria cause disease. *The Journal of Infectious Diseases* 1999;179 Suppl 2:S331-S337.

10. Centers for Disease Control and Prevention (CDC). Outbreaks of gastroenteritis associated with noroviruses on cruise ships — United States 2002. *Morbidity and Mortality Weekly Report* 2002;51:1112-1114.

11. Sanchez JL, Gelnett J, Petruccelli BP, Defraites RF, Taylor DN. Diarrheal disease incidence and morbidity among United States military personnel during

short-term missions overseas. *American Journal of Tropical Medicine and Hygiene* 1998;58:299-304.

12. Minooee A, Rickman LS. Infectious diseases on cruise ships. *Clinical Infectious Diseases* 1999;29:737-743.

13. Daniels NA, Neimann J, Karpati A, Parashar UD, Greene KD, Wells JG, Srivastava A, Tauxe RV, Mintz ED, Quick R. Traveler's diarrhea at sea: Three outbreaks of waterborne enterotoxigenic *Escherichia coli* on cruise ships. *The Journal of Infectious Diseases* 2000;181:1491-1495.

14. Lawrence DN. Outbreaks of gastrointestinal diseases on cruise ships: Lessons from three decades of progress. *Current Infectious Disease Reports* 2004; 6:115-123.

15. Addiss DG, Tauxe RV, Bernard KW. Chronic diarrhoeal illness in US Peace Corps volunteers. *International Journal of Epidemiology* 1990;19:217-218.

16. Clarke SC. Diarrhoeagenic *Escherichia coli*—an emerging problem? *Diagnostic Microbiology and Infectious Diseases* 2001;41:93-98.

17. Adachi JA, Jiang ZD, Mathewson JJ, Verenkar MP, Thompson S, Martinez-Sandoval F, Steffen R, Ericsson CD, DuPont HL. Enteroaggregative *Escherichia coli* as a major etiologic agent in traveler's diarrhea in 3 regions of the world. *Clinical Infectious Diseases* 2001;32:1706-1709.

18. Sanders JW, Isenbarger DW, Walz SE, Pang LW, Scott DA, Tamminga C, Oyofo BA, Hewitson WC, Sanchez JL, Pitarangsi C, et al. An observational clinic-based study of diarrheal illness in deployed United States military personnel in Thailand: Presentation and outcome of Campylobacter infection. *American Journal of Tropical Medicine and Hygiene* 2002;67:533-538.

19. Ericsson CD. Travelers' diarrhea. Epidemiology, prevention, and self-treatment. *Infectious Disease Clinics of North America* 1998;12:285-303.

20. Scarpignato C, Rampal P. Prevention and treatment of traveler's diarrhea: A clinical pharmacological approach. *Chemotherapy* 1995;41 Suppl 1:48-81.

21. McFarland LV. Microecologic approaches for traveler's diarrhea, antibiotic-associated diarrhea, and acute pediatric diarrhea. *Current Gastroenterology Reports* 1999;1:301-307.

22. McFarland LV. A review of the evidence of health claims for biotherapeutic agents. *Microbial Ecology in Health and Disease* 2000;12:65-76.

23. McFarland LV. Normal flora: Diversity and functions. *Microbial Ecology in Health and Disease* 2000;12:193-207.

24. Elmer GW. Probiotics: "living drugs". *American Journal of Health-System Pharmacy* 2001;58:1101-1109.

25. Kollaritsch H, Holst H, Grobara P, Wiedermann G [Prevention of traveler's diarrhea with *Saccharomyces boulardii*. Results of a placebo controlled double-blind study]. *Fortschritte der Medizin* 1993;111:152-156.

26. Kollaritsch, H, Kremsner P, Wiedermann G, and Scheiner O. Prevention of traveller's diarrhea: Comparison of different non-antibiotic preparations. *Travel Medicine International* 1989;79-18.

27. Katelaris PH, Salam I, Farthing MJ. Lactobacilli to prevent traveler's diarrhea? *The New England Journal of Medicine* 1995;333:1360-1361.

28. Oksanen PJ, Salminen S, Saxelin M, Hamalainen P, Ihantolavormisto A, Muurasniemiisoviita L, Nikkari S, Oksanen T, Porsti I, Salminen E, Siitonen S, Stuckey H, Toppila A, Vapaatalo H. Prevention of travelers diarrhea by *Lactobacillus* GG. *Annals of Medicine* 1990;22:53-56.

29. Hilton E, Kolakowski P, Singer C, Smith M. Efficacy of *Lactobacillus* GG as a diarrheal preventive in travelers. *Journal of Travel Medicine* 1997;4:41-43.

30. dios Pozo-Olano J, Warram JH, Jr., Gomez RG, Cavazos MG. Effect of a lactobacilli preparation on traveler's diarrhea. A randomized, double blind clinical trial. *Gastroenterology* 1978;74:829-830.

31. Black F, Anderson P, Orskov J, Gaarslev K, Laulund S. Prophylactic efficacy of Lactobacilli on travellers' diarrhea. *Travel Medicine* 1989;7:333-335.

32. Klein SM, Elmer GW, McFarland LV, Surawicz CM, Levy RH. Recovery and elimination of the biotherapeutic agent, *Saccharomyces boulardii*, in healthy human volunteers. *Pharmaceutical Research* 1993;10:1615-1619.

33. Kollaritsch, H, Stemberger, H, Ambrosch, P Ambrosch F, and Widermann, G. Prophylaxe des Reisendiarrhoe mit einem Lyophilisat von *Lactobacillus acidophilus* [Prophylaxis of traveler's diarrhea using a *Lactobacillus acidophilus* lyophilizate]. Gemeinsame Tagung des Deutschen Tropenmedizinischen Gesellschaft und der Osterreichischen Gesellschaft fur Tropenmedizin und Parasitologie; 1983; Meeting Abstract 92.

34. Goldin BR. Health benefits of probiotics. *The British Journal of Nutrition* 1998;80:S203-S207.

35. Ariano RE, Zhanel GG, Harding GK. The role of anion-exchange resins in the treatment of antibiotic-associated pseudomembranous colitis. *Canadian Medical Association Journal* 1990;142:1049-1051.

36. Wistrom J, Norrby R. Antibiotic prophylaxis of travellers' diarrhoea. *Scandinavian Journal of Infectious Diseases* 1990;70:111-129.

37. Adachi JA, Ericsson CD, Jiang ZD, DuPont MW, Martinez-Sandoval F, Knirsch C, DuPont HL. Azithromycin found to be comparable to levofloxacin for the treatment of US travelers with acute diarrhea acquired in Mexico. *Clinical Infectious Diseases* 2003;37:1165-1171.

38. DuPont HL, Ericsson CD, Mathewson JJ, Palazzini E, DuPont MW, Jiang ZD, Mosavi A, de la Cabada FJ. Rifaximin: A nonabsorbed antimicrobial in the therapy of travelers' diarrhea. *Digestion* 1998;59:708-714.

39. McFarland LV, Bauwens JE, Melcher SA, Surawicz CM, Greenberg RN, Elmer GW. Ciprofloxacin-associated *Clostridium difficile* disease. *Lancet* 1995; 346:977-978.

40. Bruns R, Raedsch R. Therapy of traveller's diarrhea. *Medizinische Welt* 1995;46:591-596.

41. Kirchhelle A, Fruhwein N, Toburen D. Treatment of persistent diarrhea with *S. boulardii* in returning travelers. Results of a prospective study. *Fortschritte der Medizin* 1996;114:136-140.

42. Shornikova AV, Casas IA, Mykkanen H, Salo E, Vesikari T. Bacteriotherapy with *Lactobacillus reuteri* in rotavirus gastroenteritis. *The Pediatric Infectious Disease Journal* 1997;16:1103-1107.

43. Guandalini S, Pensabene L, Zikri MA, Dias JA, Casali LG, Hoekstra H, Kolacek S, Massar K, Micetic-Turk D, Papadopoulou A, et al. *Lactobacillus* GG administered in oral rehydration solution to children with acute diarrhea: A multicenter European trial. *Journal of Pediatric Gastroenterology and Nutrition* 2000; 30:54-60.

Chapter 3

1. Van Niel CW, Feudtner C, Garrison MM, Christakis DA. Lactobacillus therapy for acute infectious diarrhea in children: A meta-analysis. *Pediatrics* 2002; 109:678-684.

2. Ribeiro H, Jr. Diarrheal disease in a developing nation. *American Journal of Gastroenterology* 2000;95:S14-S15.

3. McFarland LV, Brandmarker SA, Guandalini S. Pediatric *Clostridium difficile*: A phantom menace or clinical reality? *Journal of Pediatric Gastroenterology and Nutrition* 2000;31:220-231.

4. McFarland LV. Normal flora: Diversity and functions. *Microbial Ecology in Health and Disease* 2000;12:193-207.

5. McFarland LV, Surawicz CM, Greenberg RN, Bowen KE, Melcher SA, Mulligan ME. Possible role of cross-transmission between neonates and mothers with recurrent *Clostridium difficile* infections. *American Journal of Infection Control* 1999;27:301-303.

6. Delmee M, Verellen G, Avesani V, Francois G. *Clostridium difficile* in neonates: Serogrouping and epidemiology. *European Journal of Pediatrics* 1988; 147:36-40.

7. Larson HE, Barclay FE, Honour P, Hill ID. Epidemiology of *Clostridium difficile* in infants. *The Journal of Infectious Diseases* 1982;146:727-733.

8. Zwiener RJ, Belknap WM, Quan R. Severe pseudomembranous enterocolitis in a child: Case report and literature review. *The Pediatric Infectious Disease Journal* 1989;8:876-882.

9. Qualman SJ, Petric M, Karmali MA, Smith CR, Hamilton SR. *Clostridium difficile* invasion and toxin circulation in fatal pediatric pseudomembranous colitis. *American Journal of Clinical Pathology* 1990;94:410-416.

10. Noerr B. Current controversies in the understanding of necrotizing enterocolitis. Part 1. *Advances in Neonatal Care* 2003;3:107-120.

11. Cetina-Sauri G, Sierra Basto G. Evaluation therapeutique de *Saccharomyces boulardii* chez des enfants sourffrant de diarrhee aigue. *Annales de Pédiatrie* 1994;41:397-400.

12. Chapoy P. Treatment of acute infantile diarrhea: Controlled trial of *Saccharomyces boulardii*. *Annales de Pediatrie (Paris)* 1985;32:561-563.

13. Chouraqui J, Dietsch C, Musial H, et al. *Saccharomyces boulardii* in the management of toddler diarrhea: A double blind-placebo controlled study. *Journal of Pediatric Gastroenterology and Nutrition* 1995;20:463-465.

14. Boulloche J, Mouterde O, and Mallet E. Management of acute diarrhea in infants and toddlers: Controlled study of the antidiarrheal efficacy of killed *Lactobacillus acidophilus* (LB strain) versus placebo and a reference agent (loperamide). *Annales de Pédiatrie* 1994;41:457-463.

15. Simakachorn N, Pichaipat V, Rithipornpaisarn P, Kongkaew C, Tongpradit P, Varavithya W. Clinical evaluation of the addition of lyophilized, heat-killed *Lactobacillus acidophilus* LB to oral rehydration therapy in the treatment of acute diarrhea in children. *Journal of Pediatric Gastroenterology and Nutrition* 2000; 30:68-72.

16. Shornikova AV, Casas IA, Isolauri E, Mykkanen H, Vesikari T. *Lactobacillus reuteri* as a therapeutic agent in acute diarrhea in young children. *Journal of Pediatric Gastroenterology and Nutrition* 1997;24:399-404.

17. Shornikova AV, Casas IA, Mykkanen H, Salo E, Vesikari T. Bacteriotherapy with *Lactobacillus reuteri* in rotavirus gastroenteritis. *The Pediatric Infectious Disease Journal* 1997;16:1103-1107.

18. Pedone CA, Bernabeu AO, Postaire ER, Bouley CF, Reinert P. The effect of supplementation with milk fermented by *Lactobacillus casei* (strain DN-114 001) on acute diarrhoea in children attending day care centres. *International Journal of Clinical Practice* 1999;53:179-184.

19. Buts JP, Corthier G, Delmee M. *Saccharomyces boulardii* for *Clostridium difficile*-associated enteropathies in infants. *Journal of Pediatric Gastroenterology and Nutrition* 1993;16:419-425.

20. Costa-Ribeiro H, Ribeiro TC, Mattos AP, Valois SS, Neri DA, Almeida P, Cerqueira CM, Ramos E, Young RJ, Vanderhoof JA. Limitations of probiotic therapy in acute, severe dehydrating diarrhea. *Journal of Pediatric Gastroenterology and Nutrition* 2003;36:112-115.

21. Guandalini S, Pensabene L, Zikri MA, Dias JA, Casali LG, Hoekstra H, Kolacek S, Massar K, Micetic-Turk D, Papadopoulou A, et al. *Lactobacillus* GG administered in oral rehydration solution to children with acute diarrhea: A multicenter European trial. *Journal of Pediatric Gastroenterology and Nutrition* 2000; 30:54-60.

22. Guarino A, Canani RB, Spagnuolo MI, Albano F, Di Benedetto L. Oral bacterial therapy reduces the duration of symptoms and of viral excretion in children with mild diarrhea. *Journal of Pediatric Gastroenterology and Nutrition* 1997;25: 516-519.

23. Isolauri E, Juntunen M, Rautanen T, Sillanaukee P, Koivula T. A human Lactobacillus strain (*Lactobacillus casei* sp strain GG) promotes recovery from acute diarrhea in children. *Pediatrics* 1991;88:90-97.

24. Isolauri E, Kaila M, Mykkanen H, Ling WH, Salminen S. Oral bacteriotherapy for viral gastroenteritis. *Digestive Diseases and Sciences* 1994;39:2595-2600.

25. Kaila M, Isolauri E, Soppi E, Virtanen E, Laine S, Arvilommi H. Enhancement of the circulating antibody secreting cell response in human diarrhea by a human Lactobacillus strain. *Pediatric Research* 1992;32:141-144.

26. Majamaa H, Isolauri E, Saxelin M, Vesikari T. Lactic acid bacteria in the treatment of acute rotavirus gastroenteritis. *Journal of Pediatric Gastroenterology and Nutrition* 1995;20:333-338.

27. Pant AR, Graham SM, Allen SJ, Harikul S, Sabchareon A, Cuevas L, Hart CA. *Lactobacillus* GG and acute diarrhoea in young children in the tropics. *Journal of Tropical Pediatrics* 1996;42:162-165.

28. Raza S, Graham SM, Allen SJ, Sultana S, Cuevas L, Hart CA. *Lactobacillus* GG promotes recovery from acute nonbloody diarrhea in Pakistan. *The Pediatric Infectious Disease Journal* 1995;14:107-111.

29. Shornikova AV, Isolauri E, Burkanova L, Lukovnikova S, Vesikari T. A trial in the Karelian Republic of oral rehydration and *Lactobacillus* GG for treatment of acute diarrhoea. *Acta Paediatrica* 1997;86:460-465.

30. Chicoine L, Joncas JH. [Use of lactic enzymes in non–bacterial gastroenteritis]. *L'unión médicale du Canada* 1973;102:1114-1115.

31. Pearce JL, Hamilton JR. Controlled trial of orally administered lactobacilli in acute infantile diarrhea. *The Journal of Pediatrics* 1974;84:261-262.

32. Kaila M, Isolauri E, Saxelin M, Arvilommi H, Vesikari T. Viable versus inactivated lactobacillus strain GG in acute rotavirus diarrhoea. *Archives of Disease in Childhood* 1995;72:51-53.

33. Biller JA, Katz AJ, Flores AF, Buie TM, Gorbach SL. Treatment of recurrent *Clostridium difficile* colitis with *Lactobacillus* GG. *Journal of Pediatric Gastroenterology and Nutrition* 1995;21:224-226.

34. Lee MC, Lin LH, Hung KL, Wu HY. Oral bacterial therapy promotes recovery from acute diarrhea in children. *Acta Paediatrica Taiwanica* 2001; 42:301-305.

35. Rosenfeldt V, Michaelsen KF, Jakobsen M, Larsen CN, Moller PL, Pedersen P, Tvede M, Weyrehter H, Valerius NH, Paerregaard A. Effect of probiotic Lactobacillus strains in young children hospitalized with acute diarrhea. *The Pediatric Infectious Disease Journal* 2002;21:411-416.

36. Rosenfeldt V, Michaelsen KF, Jakobsen M, Larsen CN, Moller PL, Tvede M, Weyrehter H, Valerius NH, Paerregaard A. Effect of probiotic Lactobacillus strains on acute diarrhea in a cohort of nonhospitalized children attending day care centers. *The Pediatric Infectious Disease Journal* 2002;21:417-419.

37. Ruiz-Palacios G, Guerrero M, Tuz-Dzib F. Feeding a *Lactobacillus-reuteri*-containing probiotic drink for prevention of infantile diarrhea. *Microbial Ecology in Health and Disease* 1999;11:189.

38. Pedone CA, Arnaud CC, Postaire ER, Bouley CF, Reinert P. Multicentric study of the effect of milk fermented by *Lactobacillus casei* on the incidence of diarrhoea. *International Journal of Clinical Practice* 2000;54:568-571.

39. Szajewska H, Kotowska M, Mrukowicz JZ, Armanska M, Mikolajczyk W. Efficacy of *Lactobacillus* GG in prevention of nosocomial diarrhea in infants. *Journal of Pediatrics* 2001;138:361-365.

40. Vanderhoof JA, Whitney DB, Antonson DL, Hanner TL, Lupo JV, Young RJ. *Lactobacillus* GG in the prevention of antibiotic-associated diarrhea in children. *The Journal of Pediatrics* 1999;135:564-568.

41. Saavedra JM, Bauman NA, Oung I, Perman JA, Yolken RH. Feeding of *Bifidobacterium bifidum* and *Streptococcus thermophilus* to infants in-hospital for prevention of diarrhea and shedding of rotavirus. *Lancet* 1994;344:1046-1049.

42. Hoyos AB. Reduced incidence of necrotizing enterocolitis associated with enteral administration of *Lactobacillus acidophilus* and *Bifidobacterium infantis* to neonates in an intensive care unit. *International Journal of Infectious Diseases* 1999;3:197-202.

43. Oberhelman RA, Gilman EH, Sheen P, Taylor DN, Black RE, Cabrera L, Lescano AG, Meza R, Madico G. A placebo-controlled trial of *Lactobacillus* GG to prevent diarrhea in undernourished Peruvian children. *Journal of Pediatrics* 1999; 134:15-20.

44. Buydens P, Debeuckelaere S. Efficacy of SF 68 in the treatment of acute diarrhea. A placebo-controlled trial. *Scandinavian Journal of Gastroenterology* 1996; 31:887-891.

45. Mitra AK, Rabbani GH. A double-blind, controlled trial of bioflorin (*Streptococcus faecium* SF68) in adults with acute diarrhea due to *Vibrio cholerae* and enterotoxigenic *Escherichia coli. Gastroenterology* 1990;99:1149-1152.

46. Wunderlich PF, Braun L, Fumagalli I, D'Apuzzo V, Heim F, Karly M, Lodi R, Politta G, Vonbank F, Zeltner L. Double-blind report on the efficacy of lactic-acid-producing Enterococcus SF68 in the prevention of antibiotic-associated diarrhoea and in the treatment of acute diarrhoea. *The Journal of International Medical Research* 1989;17:333-338.

47. Hochter W, Chase D, Hagenhoff G. *Saccharomyces boulardii* bei akuter Erwachsendndiarrhoe. [Saccharomyces boulardii in treatment of acute adult diarrhea]. *Münchener Medizinische Wochenschrift* 1990;132:188-192.

48. Saint-Marc T, Blehaut H, Musial C, Touraine J. AIDS-related diarrhea: A double-blind trial of *Saccharomyces boulardii. La Semaine des Hôpitaux de Paris* 1995;71:735-741.

49. Elmer GW, Moyer KA, Vega R, Surawicz CM, Collier AC, Hooton TM, McFarland LV. Evaluation of *Saccharomyces boulardii* for patients with HIV-related chronic diarrhea and in healthy volunteers receiving antifungals. *Microecology and Therapy* 1995;25:157-171.

50. Mansour-Ghanaei F, Dehbashi N, Yazdanparast K, Shafaghi A. Efficacy of *Saccharomyces boulardii* with antibiotics in acute amoebiasis. *World Journal of Gastroenterology* 2003;9:1832-1833.

51. McFarland LV, Elmer GW, McFarland M. Meta-analysis of probiotics for the prevention and treatment of acute pediatric diarrhea. *International Journal of Probiotics and Prebiotics.* 2006;1:63-76.

52. Szajewska H, Ruszczynski M, Radzikowski A. Probiotics in the prevention of antibiotic-associated diarrhea in children: A meta-analysis of randomized controlled trials. *Journal of Pediatrics* 2006;149:367-372.

53. Johnston BC, Supina AL, Vohra S. Probiotics for pediatric antibiotic-associated diarrhea: A meta-analysis of randomized placebo-controlled trials. *Canadian Medical Association Journal* 2006;175:377-83.

54. Sazawal S, Hiremath G, Dhinga U, Malik P, Deb S, Black RE. Efficacy of probiotics in prevention of acute diarrhea: A meta-analysis of masked, randomized, placebo-controlled trials. *Lancet Infectious Diseases* 2006;6:374-82.

Chapter 4

1. Winston DJ, Ho WG, Bruckner DA, Champlin RE. Beta-lactam antibiotic therapy in febrile granulocytopenic patients. A randomized trial comparing cefo-

perazone plus piperacillin, ceftazidime plus piperacillin, and imipenem alone. *Annals of Internal Medicine* 1991;115:849-859.

2. Surawicz CM, Elmer GW, Speelman P, McFarland LV, Chinn J, Vanbelle G. Prevention of antibiotic-associated diarrhea by *Saccharomyces boulardii*—A prospective-study. *Gastroenterology* 1989;96:981-988.

3. Adam J, Barret A, Barret-Bellet E, et al. Controlled double-blind clinical trails of Ultra-Levure. Multicentre study of 25 physicians in 388 cases. *Gazette Medicale de France* 1996;84:2072-2078.

4. McFarland LV, Surawicz CM, Greenberg RN, Elmer GW, Moyer KA, Melcher SA, Bowen KE, Cox JL. Prevention of beta-lactam-associated diarrhea by *Saccharomyces boulardii* compared with placebo. *American Journal of Gastroenterology* 1995;90:439-448.

5. de Barbeyrac B, Guinet R, Quentin C, Cantet P, Bebear C. *Clostridium difficile* and its cytotoxin in diarrhoeic stools of hospitalized patients. Toxigenic potential of the isolates. *Annales de Biologie Clinque* 1989;47:67-70.

6. Hutin Y, Casin I, Lesprit P, Welker Y, Decazes JM, Lagrange P, Modai J, Molina JM. Prevalence of and risk factors for *Clostridium difficile* colonization at admission to an infectious diseases ward. *Clinical Infectious Diseases* 1997;24: 920-924.

7. Thamlikitkul V, Danpakdi K, Chokloikaew S. Incidence of diarrhea and *Clostridium difficile* toxin in stools from hospitalized patients receiving clindamycin, beta-lactams, or nonantibiotic medications. *Journal of Clinical Gastroenterology* 1996;22:161-163.

8. Bulstrode NW, Bradbury AW, Barrett S, Stansby G, Mansfield AO, Nicolaides AN, Wolfe JH. *Clostridium difficile* colitis after aortic surgery. *European Journal of Vascular and Endovascular Surgery* 1997;14:217-220.

9. Dutta P, Niyogi SK, Mitra U, Rasaily R, Bhattacharya MK, Chakraborty S, Mitra A. *Clostridium difficile* in antibiotic associated pediatric diarrhea. *Indian Pediatrics* 1994;31:121-126.

10. Brown E, Talbot GH, Axelrod P, Provencher M, Hoegg C. Risk factors for *Clostridium difficile* toxin-associated diarrhea. *Infection Control and Hospital Epidemiology* 1990;11:283-290.

11. Lai KK, Melvin ZS, Menard MJ, Kotilainen HR, Baker S. *Clostridium difficile*-associated diarrhea: Epidemiology, risk factors, and infection control. *Infection Control and Hospital Epidemiology* 1997;18:628-632.

12. James AH, Katz VL, Dotters DJ, Rogers RG. *Clostridium difficile* infection in obstetric and gynecologic patients. *The Southern Medical Journal* 1997;90:889-892.

13. McFarland LV, Mulligan ME, Kwok RY, Stamm WE. Nosocomial acquisition of *Clostridium difficile* infection. *The New England Journal of Medicine* 1989;320:204-210.

14. Knobel H, Salvado M, Segura C. [Clostridium difficile and diarrhea associated with the use of antibiotics in the origin of nosocomial and community-acquired diarrhea]. *Enfermedades Infecciosas y Microbiología Clínica* 1996;14:96-100.

15. Levy DG, Stergachis A, McFarland LV, Van Vorst K, Graham DJ, Johnson ES, Park BJ, Shatin D, Clouse JC, Elmer GW. Antibiotics and *Clostridium difficile* diarrhea in the ambulatory care setting. *Clinical Therapeutics* 2000;22:91-102.

16. Hirschhorn LR, Trnka Y, Onderdonk A, Lee ML, Platt R. Epidemiology of community-acquired *Clostridium difficile*-associated diarrhea. *The Journal of Infectious Diseases* 1994;169:127-133.

17. McFarland LV. Epidemiology, risk factors and treatments for antibiotic-associated diarrhea. *Digestive Diseases* 1998;16:292-307.

18. McFarland L. Normal flora: Diversity and functions. *Microbial Ecology in Health and Disease* 2000;12:193-207.

19. Surawicz CM, McFarland LV. Pseudomembranous colitis: Causes and cures. *Digestion* 1999;60:91-100.

20. McFarland LV. Epidemiology of infectious and iatrogenic nosocomial diarrhea in a cohort of general medicine patients. *American Journal of Infection Control* 1995;23:295-305.

21. Lima NL, Guerrant RL, Kaiser DL, Germanson T, Farr BM. A retrospective cohort study of nosocomial diarrhea as a risk factor for nosocomial infection. *The Journal of Infectious Diseases* 1990;161:948-952.

22. McFarland LV. A review of the evidence of health claims for biotherapeutic agents. *Microbial Ecology in Health and Disease* 2000;12:65-76.

23. Elmer GW, Surawicz CM, McFarland LV. Biotherapeutic agents. A neglected modality for the treatment and prevention of selected intestinal and vaginal infections. *Journal of American Medical Association* 1996;275:870-876.

24. Cremonini F, Di Caro S, Nista EC, Bartolozzi F, Capelli G, Gasbarrini G, Gasbarrini A. Meta-analysis: The effect of probiotic administration on antibiotic-associated diarrhoea. *Alimentary Pharmacology and Therapeutics* 2002;16:1461-1467.

25. D'Souza AL, Rajkumar C, Cooke J, Bulpitt CJ. Probiotics in prevention of antibiotic associated diarrhoea: Meta-analysis. *British Medical Journal* 2002;324:1361.

26. Seki H, Shiohara M, Matsumura T, Miyagawa N, Tanaka M, Komiyama A, Kurata S. Prevention of antibiotic-associated diarrhea in children by *Clostridium butyricum* MIYAIRI. *Pediatrics International* 2003;45:86-90.

27. Szajewska H, Kotowska M, Mrukowicz JZ, Armanska M, Mikolajczyk W. Efficacy of *Lactobacillus* GG in prevention of nosocomial diarrhea in infants. *Journal of Pediatrics* 2001;138:361-365.

28. Thomas MR, Litin SC, Osmon DR, Corr AP, Weaver AL, Lohse CM. Lack of effect of *Lactobacillus* GG on antibiotic-associated diarrhea: A randomized, placebo-controlled trial. *Mayo Clinic Proceedings* 2001;76:883-889.

29. Arvola T, Laiho K, Torkkeli S, Mykkanen H, Salminen S, Maunula L, Isolauri E. Prophylactic *Lactobacillus* GG reduces antibiotic-associated diarrhea in children with respiratory infections: A randomized study. *Pediatrics* 1999;104:e64.

30. Vanderhoof JA, Whitney DB, Antonson DL, Hanner TL, Lupo JV, Young RJ. *Lactobacillus* GG in the prevention of antibiotic-associated diarrhea in children. *The Journal of Pediatrics* 1999;135:564-568.

31. Lewis SJ, Potts LF, Barry RE. The lack of therapeutic effect of *Saccharomyces boulardii* in the prevention of antibiotic-related diarrhoea in elderly patients. *The Journal of Infection* 1998;36:171-174.

32. Kotowska M, Albrecht P, Szajewska H. *Saccharomyces boulardii* in the prevention of antibiotic-associated diarrhoea in children: A randomized double-

blind placebo-controlled trial. *Alimentary Pharmacology and Therapeutics* 2005; 21:583-590.

33. Tankanow RM, Ross MB, Ertel IJ, Dickinson DG, McCormick LS, Garfinkel JF. A double-blind, placebo-controlled study of the efficacy of Lactinex in the prophylaxis of amoxicillin-induced diarrhea. *Drug Intelligence and Clinical Pharmacy* 1990;24:382-384.

34. Gotz V, Romankiewicz JA, Moss J, Murray HW. Prophylaxis against ampicillin-associated diarrhea with a lactobacillus preparation. *American Journal of Hospital Pharmacy* 1979;36:754-757.

35. Wunderlich PF, Braun L, Fumagalli I, D'Apuzzo V, Heim F, Karly M, Lodi R, Politta G, Vonbank F, Zeltner L. Double-blind report on the efficacy of lactic acid-producing Enterococcus SF68 in the prevention of antibiotic-associated diarrhoea and in the treatment of acute diarrhoea. *The Journal of International Medical research* 1989;17:333-338.

36. Szajewska H, Mrukowicz JZ. Probiotics in the treatment and prevention of acute infectious diarrhea in infants and children: A systematic review of published randomized, double-blind, placebo-controlled trials. *Journal of Pediatric Gastroenterology and Nutrition* 2001;33 Suppl 2:S17-S25.

37. McFarland LV, Surawicz CM, Greenberg RN, Bowen KE, Melcher SA, Mulligan ME. Possible role of cross-transmission between neonates and mothers with recurrent *Clostridium difficile* infections. *American Journal of Infection Control* 1999;27:301-303.

38. Fekety R. Guidelines for the diagnosis and management of *Clostridium difficile*-associated diarrhea and colitis. American College of Gastroenterology, Practice Parameters Committee. *American Journal of Gastroenterology* 1997;92: 739-750.

39. Fekety R, McFarland LV, Surawicz CM, Greenberg RN, Elmer GW, Mulligan ME. Recurrent *Clostridium difficile* diarrhea: Characteristics of and risk factors for patients enrolled in a prospective, randomized, double-blinded trial. *Clinical Infectious Diseases* 1997;24:324-333.

40. McFarland LV, Surawicz CM, Rubin M, Fekety R, Elmer GW, Greenberg RN. Recurrent *Clostridium difficile* disease: Epidemiology and clinical characteristics. *Infection Control and Hospital Epidemiology* 1999;20:43-50.

41. Gerding DN. Is there a relationship between vancomycin-resistant enterococcal infection and *Clostridium difficile* infection? *Clinical Infectious Diseases* 1997;25 Suppl 2:S206-S210.

42. Kofsky P, Rosen L, Reed J, Tolmie M, Ufberg D. *Clostridium difficile*—a common and costly colitis. *Diseases of the Colon and Rectum* 1991;34:244-248.

43. Olson MM, Shanholtzer CJ, Lee JT, Jr., Gerding DN. Ten years of prospective *Clostridium difficile*-associated disease surveillance and treatment at the Minneapolis VA Medical Center, 1982–1991. *Infection Control and Hospital Epidemiology* 1994;15:371-381.

44. Surawicz CM, McFarland LV. Pseudomembranous colitis caused by *Clostridium difficile*. *Current Treatment Options in Gastroenterology* 2000;3:203-210.

45. Wenisch C, Parschalk B, Hasenhundl M, Hirschl AM, Graninger W. Comparison of vancomycin, teicoplanin, metronidazole, and fusidic acid for the treatment

of *Clostridium difficile*-associated diarrhea. *Clinical Infectious Diseases* 1996; 22:813-818.

46. McFarland LV, Surawicz CM, Greenberg RN, Fekety R, Elmer GW, Moyer KA, Melcher SA, Bowen KE, Cox JL, Noorani Z,. A randomized placebo-controlled trial of *Saccharomyces boulardii* in combination with standard antibiotics for *Clostridium difficile* disease. *Journal of American Medical Association* 1994; 271:1913-1918.

47. Surawicz CM, McFarland LV, Greenberg RN, Rubin M, Fekety R, Mulligan ME, Garcia RJ, Brandmarker S, Bowen K, Borjal D, Elmer GW. The search for a better treatment for recurrent *Clostridium difficile* disease: Use of high-dose vancomycin combined with *Saccharomyces boulardii*. *Clinical Infectious Diseases* 2000;31:1012-1017.

48. McFarland LV, Elmer GW, Surawicz CM. Breaking the cycle: Treatment strategies for 163 cases of recurrent *Clostridium difficile* disease. *American Journal of Gastroenterology* 2002;97:1769-1775.

49. Pochapin M. The effect of probiotics on *Clostridium difficile* diarrhea. *American Journal of Gastroenterology* 2000;95:S11-S13.

50. Wullt M, Hagslatt ML, Odenholt I. *Lactobacillus plantarum* 299v for the treatment of recurrent *Clostridium difficile*-associated diarrhoea: A double-blind, placebo-controlled trial. *Scandinavian Journal of Infectious Diseases* 2003;35:365-367.

51. Surawicz CM, McFarland LV, Elmer G, Chinn J. Treatment of recurrent *Clostridium difficile* colitis with vancomycin and *Saccharomyces boulardii*. *American Journal of Gastroenterology* 1989;84:1285-1287.

52. Buts JP, Corthier G, Delmee M. *Saccharomyces boulardii* for *Clostridium difficile*-associated enteropathies in infants. *Journal of Pediatric Gastroenterology and Nutrition* 1993;16:419-425.

53. Gorbach SL, Chang TW, Goldin B. Successful treatment of relapsing *Clostridium difficile* colitis with *Lactobacillus* GG. *Lancet* 1987;2:1519.

54. Biller JA, Katz AJ, Flores AF, Buie TM, Gorbach SL. Treatment of recurrent *Clostridium difficile* colitis with *Lactobacillus* GG. *Journal of Pediatric Gastroenterology and Nutrition* 1995;21:224-226.

55. Bennett R, Gorbach S, Goldin R, Chang T. Treatment of relapsing *Clostridium difficile* diarrhea with *Lactobacillus* GG. *Nutrition Today* 1996;31:S35-S38.

56. Schellenberg D, Bonington A, Champion CM, Lancaster R, Webb S, Main J. Treatment of *Clostridium difficile* diarrhoea with brewer's yeast. *Lancet* 1994;343: 171-172.

57. Kimmey MB, Elmer GW, Surawicz CM, McFarland LV. Prevention of further recurrences of *Clostridium difficile* colitis with *Saccharomyces boulardii*. *Digestive Diseases and Sciences* 1990;35:897-901.

58. Hassett J, Meyers S, McFarland L, Mulligan ME. Recurrent *Clostridium difficile* infection in a patient with selective IgG1 deficiency treated with intravenous immune globulin and *Saccharomyces boulardii*. *Clinical Infectious Diseases* 1995;20 Suppl 2:S266-S268.

59. McFarland LV. Meta-analysis of probiotics for the prevention of antibiotic associated diarrhea and the treatment of *Clostridium difficile* disease. *American Journal of Gastroenterology* 2006;101:812-22.

60. Sazawal S, Hiremath G, Dhinga U, Malik P, Deb S, Black RE. Efficacy of probiotics in prevention of acute diarrhea: A meta-analysis of masked, randomized, placebo-controlled trials. *Lancet Infectious Diseases* 2006;6:374-82.

61. Szajewska H, Mrukovicz J. Meta-analysis: Non-pathogenic yeast *Saccharomyces boulardii* in the prevention of antibiotic-associated diarrhea. *Alimentary Pharmacology and Therapy*. 2005;22:365-72.

Chapter 5

1. Van Kessel K, Assefi N, Marrazzo J, Eckert L. Common complementary and alternative therapies for yeast vaginitis and bacterial vaginosis: A systematic review. *Obstetrical and Gynecological Survey* 2003;58:351-358.

2. Sewankambo N, Gray RH, Wawer MJ, Paxton L, McNaim D, Wabwire-Mangen F, Serwadda D, Li C, Kiwanuka N, Hillier SL, et al. HIV-1 infection associated with abnormal vaginal flora morphology and bacterial vaginosis. *Lancet* 1997; 350:546-550.

3. van de Wijgert JH, Mason PR, Gwanzura L, Mbizvo MT, Chirenje ZM, Iliff V, Shiboski S, Padian NS. Intravaginal practices, vaginal flora disturbances, and acquisition of sexually transmitted diseases in Zimbabwean women. *The Journal of Infectious Diseases* 2000;181:587-594.

4. Jacobsson B, Pernevi P, Chidekel L, Jorgen Platz-Christensen J. Bacterial vaginosis in early pregnancy may predispose for preterm birth and postpartum endometritis. *Acta Obstetricia et Gynecologica Scandinavica* 2002;81:1006-1010.

5. Reid G, Devillard E. Probiotics for mother and child. *Journal of Clinical Gastroenterology* 2004;38:S94-S101.

6. Hillier SL, Nugent RP, Eschenbach DA, Krohn MA, Gibbs RS, Martin DH, Cotch MF, Edelman R, Pastorek JG, Rao AV, Association between bacterial vaginosis and preterm delivery of a low-birth-weight infant. The Vaginal Infections and Prematurity Study Group. *The New England Journal of Medicine* 1995;333:1737-1742.

7. Reid G, Bocking A. The potential for probiotics to prevent bacterial vaginosis and preterm labor. *American Journal of Obstetrics and Gynecology* 2003;189: 1202-1208.

8. Carey JC, Klebanoff MA, Hauth JC, Hillier SL, Thom EA, Ernest JM, Heine RP, Nugent RP, Fischer ML, Leveno KJ, et al. Metronidazole to prevent preterm delivery in pregnant women with asymptomatic bacterial vaginosis. National Institute of Child Health and Human Development Network of Maternal-Fetal Medicine Units. *The New England Journal of Medicine* 2000;342:534-540.

9. Neri A, Sabah G, Samra Z. Bacterial vaginosis in pregnancy treated with yoghurt. *Acta Obstetricia et Gynecologica Scandinavica* 1993;72:17-19.

10. Hallen A, Jarstrand C, Pahlson C. Treatment of bacterial vaginosis with lactobacilli. *Sexually Transmitted Diseases* 1992;19:146-148.

11. Parent D, Bossens M, Bayot D, Kirkpatrick C, Graf F, Wilkinson FE, Kaiser RR. Therapy of bacterial vaginosis using exogenously-applied *Lactobacilli acidophilis* and a low dose of estriol: A placebo-controlled multicentric clinical trial. *Arzneimittelforschung* 1996;46:68-73.

12. Shalev E, Battino S, Weiner E, Colodner R, Keness Y. Ingestion of yogurt containing *Lactobacillus acidophilus* compared with pasteurized yogurt as prophylaxis for recurrent candidal vaginitis and bacterial vaginosis. *Archives of Family Medicine* 1996;5:593-596.

13. Reid G, Charbonneau D, Erb J, Kochanowski B, Beuerman D, Poehner R, Bruce AW. Oral use of *Lactobacillus rhamnosus* GR-1 and *L. fermentum* RC-14 significantly alters vaginal flora: Randomized, placebo-controlled trial in 64 healthy women. FEMS *Immunology and Medical Microbiology* 2003;35:131-134.

14. Reid G, Bruce AW. Selection of Lactobacillus strains for urogenital probiotic applications. *Journal of Infectious Diseases* 2001;183:S77-S80.

15. Nyirjesy P, Weitz MV, Grody MH, Lorber B. Over-the-counter and alternative medicines in the treatment of chronic vaginal symptoms. *Obstetrics and Gynecology* 1997;90:50-53.

16. Sobell JD. Biotherapeutic agents as therapy for vaginitis. In: Elmer GW, McFarland LV, Surawicz CM, eds. *Biotherapeutic Agents and Infectious Diseases.* Totowa, New Jersey: Humana Press, 1999:221-244.

17. *The Merck Manual of Diagnosis and Therapy.* Mark H Beers and Robert R Berkow (eds) Merck and Company, Inc., Rahway, N.J. 1999.

18. Hilton E, Isenberg HD, Alperstein P, France K, Borenstein MT. Ingestion of yogurt containing *Lactobacillus acidophilus* as prophylaxis for candidal vaginitis. *Annals of Internal Medicine* 1992;116:353-357.

19. Hilton E, Rindos P, Isenberg HD. *Lactobacillus* GG vaginal suppositories and vaginitis. *Journal of Clinical Microbiology* 1995;33:1433.

20. Wagner RD, Pierson C, Warner T, Dohnalek M, Hilty M, Balish E. Probiotic effects of feeding heat-killed *Lactobacillus acidophilus* and *Lactobacillus casei* to *Candida albicans*-colonized immunodeficient mice. *Journal of Food Protection* 2000;63:638-644.

21. Pirotta M, Gunn J, Chondros P, Grover S, O'Malley P, Hurley S, Garland S. Effect of lactobacillus in preventing post-antibiotic vulvovaginal candidiasis: A randomised controlled trial. *British Medical Journal* 2004;329:548.

22. Ikaheimo R, Siitonen A, Heiskanen T, Karkkainen U, Kuosmanen P, Lipponen P, Makela PH. Recurrence of urinary tract infection in a primary care setting: Analysis of a 1-year follow-up of 179 women. *Clinical Infectious Diseases* 1996; 22:91-99.

23. Hooton TM. The current management strategies for community-acquired urinary tract infection. *Infectious Disease Clinics of North America* 2003;17:303-332.

24. Kontiokari T, Sundqvist K, Nuutinen M, Pokka T, Koskela M, Uhari M. Randomised trial of cranberry-lingonberry juice and *Lactobacillus* GG drink for the prevention of urinary tract infections in women. *British Medical Journal* 2001; 322:1571.

25. Hooton TM. Recurrent urinary tract infection in women. *International Journal of Antimicrobial Agents* 2001;17:259-268.

26. Gupta K, Stapleton AE, Hooton TM, Roberts PL, Fennell CL, Stamm WE. Inverse association of H_2O_2-producing lactobacilli and vaginal *Escherichia coli* col-

onization in women with recurrent urinary tract infections. *The Journal of Infectious Diseases* 1998;178:446-450.

27. Reid G, Servin AL, Bruce AW, Busscher HJ. Adhesion of three Lactobacillus strains to human urinary and intestinal epithelial cells. *Microbios* 1993;75:57-65.

28. Reid G, Bruce AW, McGroarty JA, Cheng KJ, Costerton JW. Is there a role for lactobacilli in prevention of urogenital and intestinal infections? *Clinical Microbiology Reviews* 1990;3:335-344.

29. Bruce AW, Reid G. Intravaginal instillation of lactobacilli for prevention of recurrent urinary tract infections. *Canadian Journal of Microbiology* 1988;34:339-343.

30. Reid G, Bruce AW, Taylor M. Influence of three-day antimicrobial therapy and lactobacillus vaginal suppositories on recurrence of urinary tract infections. *Clinical Therapeutics* 1992;14:11-16.

31. Baerheim A, Larsen E, Digranes A. Vaginal application of lactobacilli in the prophylaxis of recurrent lower urinary tract infection in women. *Scandinavian Journal of Primary Health Care* 1994;12:239-243.

Chapter 6

1. Clark E, Hoare C, Tanianis-huges J, Carlson GL, Warhurst G. Interferon gamma induces translocation of commensal *Escherichia coli* across gut epithelial cells via a lipid-raft medicated process. *Gastroenterology* 2005;128:1258-1276.

2. DeSimone EM, Lanspa SJ, Hogrefe D, Terlaje C. Management and treatment of Crohn's disease. *U S Pharmacist* 2004;29:95-102.

3. Farrell RJ, Lamont JT. Microbial factors in inflammatory bowel disease. *Gastroenterology Clinics of North America* 2002;31:41-62.

4. Kaila M, Isolauri E, Saxelin M, Arvilommi H, Vesikari T. Viable versus inactivated lactobacillus strain GG in acute rotavirus diarrhoea. *Archives of Disease in Childhood* 1995;72:51-53.

5. Qamar A, Aboudola S, Warny M, Michetti P, Pothoulakis C, Lamont JT, Kelly CP. *Saccharomyces boulardii* stimulates intestinal immunoglobulin A immune response to *Clostridium difficile* toxin A in mice. *Infection and Immunity* 2001;69: 2762-2765.

6. Schultz M, Scholmerich J, Rath HC. Rationale for probiotic and antibiotic treatment strategies in inflammatory bowel diseases. *Digestive Diseases* 2003;21: 105-128.

7. Schultz M, Veltkamp C, Dieleman LA, Grenther WB, Wyrick PB, Tonkonogy SL, Sartor RB. *Lactobacillus plantarum* 299V in the treatment and prevention of spontaneous colitis in interleukin-10-deficient mice. *Inflammatory Bowel Diseases* 2002;8:71-80.

8. Prantera C, Scribano ML, Falasco G, Andreoli A, Luzi C. Ineffectiveness of probiotics in preventing recurrence after curative resection for Crohn's disease: A randomised controlled trial with *Lactobacillus* GG. *Gut* 2002;51:405-409.

9. Schultz M, Timmer A, Herfarth HH, Sartor RB, Vanderhoof JA, Rath HC. *Lactobacillus* GG in inducing and maintaining remission of Crohn's disease. *Biomedical Chromatography Gastroenterology* 2004;4:5.

10. Plein K, Hotz J. Therapeutic effects of *Saccharomyces boulardii* on mild residual symptoms in a stable phase of Crohn's disease with special respect to chronic diarrhea—a pilot study. *Zeitschrift für Gastroenterologie* 1993;31:129-134.

11. Guslandi M, Mezzi G, Sorghi M, Testoni PA. *Saccharomyces boulardii* in maintenance treatment of Crohn's disease. *Digestive Diseases and Sciences* 2000; 45:1462-1464.

12. Malchow HA. Crohn's disease and *Escherichia coli*. A new approach in therapy to maintain remission of colonic Crohn's disease? *Journal of Clinical Gastroenterology* 1997;25:653-658.

13. Taurog JD, Richardson JA, Croft JT, Simmons WA, Zhou M, Fernandez-Sueiro JL, Balish E, Hammer RE. The germfree state prevents development of gut and joint inflammatory disease in HLA-B27 transgenic rats. *The Journal of Experimental Medicine* 1994;180:2359-2364.

14. Kwon J, Farrell R. Probiotics and inflammatory bowel disease. *BioDrugs* 2003;17:179-186.

15. *The Merck Manual of Diagnosis and Therapy*. Mark H. Beers and Robert R. Berkow (eds.) Merck and Company, Inc., Rahway, N.J. 1999.

16. Podolsky DK. Inflammatory bowel disease. *The New England Journal of Medicine* 2002;347:417-429.

17. Rembacken BJ, Snelling AM, Hawkey PM, Chalmers DM, Axon AT. Nonpathogenic *Escherichia coli* versus mesalazine for the treatment of ulcerative colitis: A randomised trial. *Lancet* 1999;354:635-639.

18. Kruis W, Schutz E, Fric P, Fixa B, Judmaier G, Stolte M. Double-blind comparison of an oral *Escherichia coli* preparation and mesalazine in maintaining remission of ulcerative colitis. *Alimentary Pharmacology and Therapeutics* 1997; 11:853-858.

19. Kruis W, Fric P, Pokrotnieks J, Lukas M, Fixa B, Kascak M, Kamm MA, Weismueller J, Beglinger C, Stolte M, Wolff C, Schulze J. Maintaining remission of ulcerative colitis with the probiotic *Escherichia coli* Nissle 1917 is as effective as with standard mesalazine. *Gut* 2004;53:1617-1623.

20. Venturi A, Gionchetti P, Rizzello F, Johansson R, Zucconi E, Brigidi P, Matteuzzi D, Campieri M. Impact on the composition of the faecal flora by a new probiotic preparation: Preliminary data on maintenance treatment of patients with ulcerative colitis. *Alimentary Pharmacology and Therapeutics* 1999;13:1103-1108.

21. Katz JA. Prevention is the best defense: Probiotic prophylaxis of pouchitis. *Gastroenterology* 2003;124:1535-1538.

22. Gionchetti P, Rizzello F, Venturi A, Brigidi P, Matteuzzi D, Bazzocchi G, Poggioli G, Miglioli M, Campieri M. Oral bacteriotherapy as maintenance treatment in patients with chronic pouchitis: A double-blind, placebo-controlled trial. *Gastroenterology* 2000;119:305-309.

23. Gionchetti P, Rizzello F, Helwig U, Venturi A, Lammers KM, Brigidi P, Vitali B, Poggioli G, Miglioli M, Campieri M. Prophylaxis of pouchitis onset with probiotic therapy: A double-blind, placebo-controlled trial. *Gastroenterology* 2003; 124:1202-1209.

24. Mimura T, Rizzello F, Helwig U, Poggioli G, Schreiber S, Talbot IC, Nicholls RJ, Gionchetti P, Campieri M, Kamm MA. Once daily high dose probiotic

therapy (VSL#3) for maintaining remission in recurrent or refractory pouchitis. *Gut* 2004;53:108-114.

25. Gosselink MP, Schouten WR, van Lieshout LM, Hop WC, Laman JD, Ruseler-van Embden JG. Delay of the first onset of pouchitis by oral intake of the probiotic strain *Lactobacillus rhamnosus* GG. *Diseases of the Colon and Rectum* 2004;47:876-884.

26. Drossman DA, Whitehead WE, Camilleri M. Irritable bowel syndrome: A technical review for practice guideline development. *Gastroenterology* 1997;112: 2120-2137.

27. Di Stefano M, Strocchi A, Malservisi S, Veneto G, Ferrieri A, Corazza GR. Non-absorbable antibiotics for managing intestinal gas production and gas-related symptoms. *Alimentary Pharmacology and Therapeutics* 2000;14:1001-1008.

28. Pimentel M, Chow EJ, Lin HC. Eradication of small intestinal bacterial overgrowth reduces symptoms of irritable bowel syndrome. *American Journal of Gastroenterology* 2000;95:3503-3506.

29. Sen S, Mullan MM, Parker TJ, Woolner JT, Tarry SA, Hunter JO. Effect of *Lactobacillus plantarum* 299v on colonic fermentation and symptoms of irritable bowel syndrome. *Digestive Diseases and Sciences* 2002;47:2615-2620.

30. Niedzielin K, Kordecki H, Birkenfeld B. A controlled, double-blind, randomized study on the efficacy of *Lactobacillus plantarum* 299V in patients with irritable bowel syndrome. *European Journal of Gastroenterology and hepatology* 2001;13:1143-1147.

31. Nobaek S, Johansson ML, Molin G, Ahrne S, Jeppsson B. Alteration of intestinal microflora is associated with reduction in abdominal bloating and pain in patients with irritable bowel syndrome. *American Journal of Gastroenterology* 2000;95:1231-1238.

32. O'Sullivan MA, O'Morain CA. Bacterial supplementation in the irritable bowel syndrome. A randomised double-blind placebo-controlled crossover study. *Digestive and Liver Disease* 2000;32:294-301.

33. Kim HJ, Camilleri M, McKinzie S, Lempke MB, Burton DD, Thomforde GM, Zinsmeister AR. A randomized controlled trial of a probiotic, VSL#3, on gut transit and symptoms in diarrhoea-predominant irritable bowel syndrome. *Alimentary Pharmacology and Therapeutics* 2003;17:895-904.

34. Bazzocchi G, Gionchetti P, Almerigi PF, Amadini C, Campieri M. Intestinal microflora and oral bacteriotherapy in irritable bowel syndrome. *Digestive and Liver Disease* 2002;34 Suppl 2:S48-S53.

35. Saggioro A. Probiotics in the treatment of irritable bowel syndrome. *Journal of Clinical Gastroenterology* 2004;38:S104-S106.

36. O'Mahony L, McCarthy J, Kelly P, Hurley G, Luo F, Chen K, O'Sullivan GC, Kiely B, Collins, JK, Shanahan F, Quigley EMM. Lactobacillus and Bifidobacterium in irritable bowel syndrome: Symptom responses and relationship to cytokine profiles. *Gastroenterology* 2005;128:541-551.

37. Burton JP, Tannock GW. Properties of porcine and yogurt lactobacilli in relation to lactose intolerance. *Journal of Dairy Science* 1997;80:2318-2324.

38. Saltzman JR, Russell RM, Golner B, Barakat S, Dallal GE, Goldin BR. A randomized trial of *Lactobacillus acidophilus* BG2FO4 to treat lactose intolerance. *American Journal of Clinical Nutrition* 1999;69:140-146.

39. Zoppi G, Cinquetti M, Luciano A, Benini A, Muner A, Bertazzoni ME. The intestinal ecosystem in chronic functional constipation. *Acta Paediatrica* 1998; 87:836-841.

40. Ouwehand AC, Lagstrom H, Suomalainen T, Salminen S. Effect of probiotics on constipation, fecal azoreductase activity and fecal mucin content in the elderly. *Annals of Nutrition and Metabolism* 2002;46:159-162.

41. Koebnick C, Wagner I, Leitzmann P, Stern U, Zunft HJ. Probiotic beverage containing *Lactobacillus casei* Shirota improves gastrointestinal symptoms in patients with chronic constipation. *Canadian Journal of Gastroenterology* 2003;17: 655-659.

Chapter 7

1. Laiho K, Ouwehand A, Salminen S, Isolauri E. Inventing probiotic functional foods for patients with allergic disease. *Annals of Allergy, Asthma and Immunology* 2002;89:75-82.

2. Strachan DP. Hay fever, hygiene, and household size. *British Medical Journal* 1989;299:1259-1260.

3. Sheikh A, Strachan DP. The hygiene theory: Fact or fiction? *Current Opinion in Otolaryngology and Head and Neck Surgery* 2004;12:232-236.

4. da Costa LR, Victora CG, Menezes AM, Barros FC. Do risk factors for childhood infections and malnutrition protect against asthma? A study of Brazilian male adolescents. *American Journal of Public Health* 2003;93:1858-1864.

5. von Mutius E, Martinez FD, Fritzsch C, Nicolai T, Reitmeir P, Thiemann HH. Skin test reactivity and number of siblings. *British Medical Journal* 1994;308:692-695.

6. Watanabe S, Narisawa Y, Arase S, Okamatsu H, Ikenaga T, Tajiri Y, Kumemura M. Differences in fecal microflora between patients with atopic dermatitis and healthy control subjects. *The Journal of Allergy and Clinical Immunology* 2003; 111:587-591.

7. Kalliomaki M, Kirjavainen P, Eerola E, Kero P, Salminen S, Isolauri E. Distinct patterns of neonatal gut microflora in infants in whom atopy was and was not developing. *The Journal of Allergy and Clinical Immunology* 2001;107:129-134.

8. Alm JS, Swartz J, Bjorksten B, Engstrand L, Engstrom J, Kuhn I, Lilja G, Mollby R, Norin E, Pershagen G, Reinders C, Wreiber K, Scheynius A. An anthroposophic lifestyle and intestinal microflora in infancy. *Pediatric Allergy and Immunology* 2002;13:402-411.

9. Alm JS, Swartz J, Lilja G, Scheynius A, Pershagen G. Atopy in children of families with an anthroposophic lifestyle. *Lancet* 1999;353:1485-1488.

10. Matricardi PM, Rosmini F, Panetta V, Ferrigno L, Bonini S. Hay fever and asthma in relation to markers of infection in the United States. *The Journal of Allergy and Clinical Immunology* 2002;110:381-387.

11. Matricardi PM, Rosmini F, Riondino S, Fortini M, Ferrigno L, Rapicetta M, Bonini S. Exposure to foodborne and orofecal microbes versus airborne viruses in relation to atopy and allergic asthma: Epidemiological study. *British Medical Journal* 2000;320:412-417.

12. *Harrison's Principles of Internal Medicine.* Deniis L. Kaspar (ed.) McGraw-Hill, New York City, N.Y. 2005.

13. *The Merck Manual of Diagnosis and Therapy.* Mark H. Beers and Robert R. Berkow (eds.) Merck and Company, Inc., Rahway, N.J. 1999.

14. Pessi T, Isolauri E, Sutas Y, Kankaanranta H, Moilanen E, Hurme M. Suppression of T-cell activation by *Lactobacillus rhamnosus* GG-degraded bovine casein. *International Immunopharmacology* 2001;1:211-218.

15. Sutas Y, Soppi E, Korhonen H, Syvaoja EL, Saxelin M, Rokka T, Isolauri E. Suppression of lymphocyte proliferation in vitro by bovine caseins hydrolyzed with *Lactobacillus casei* GG-derived enzymes. *The Journal of Allergy and Clinical Immunology* 1996;98:216-224.

16. Qamar A, Aboudola S, Warny M, Michetti P, Pothoulakis C, Lamont JT, Kelly CP. *Saccharomyces boulardii* stimulates intestinal immunoglobulin A immune response to *Clostridium difficile* toxin A in mice. *Infection and Immunity* 2001;69:2762-2765.

17. Kaila M, Isolauri E, Saxelin M, Arvilommi H, Vesikari T. Viable versus inactivated Lactobacillus strain GG in acute rotavirus diarrhoea. *Archives of Disease in Childhood* 1995;72:51-53.

18. Viljanen M, Kuitunen M, Haahtela T, Juntunen-Backman K, Korpela R, Savilahti E. Probiotic effects on faecal inflammatory markers and on faecal IgA in food allergic atopic eczema/dermatitis syndrome infants. *Pediatric Allergy and Immunology* 2005;16:65-71.

19. Laiho K, Hoppu U, Ouwehand AC, Salminen S, Isolauri E. Probiotics: Ongoing research on atopic individuals. *The British Journal of Nutrition* 2002;88 Suppl 1:S19-S27.

20. Pessi T, Sutas Y, Hurme M, Isolauri E. Interleukin-10 generation in atopic children following oral *Lactobacillus rhamnosus* GG. *Clinical and Experimental Allergy* 2000;30:1804-1808.

21. Majamaa H, Isolauri E. Probiotics: A novel approach in the management of food allergy. *The Journal of Allergy and Clinical Immunology* 1997;99:179-185.

22. Isolauri E, Arvola T, Sutas Y, Moilanen E, Salminen S. Probiotics in the management of atopic eczema. *Clinical and Experimental Allergy* 2000;30:1604-1610.

23. Kirjavainen PV, Salminen SJ, Isolauri E. Probiotic bacteria in the management of atopic disease: Underscoring the importance of viability. *Journal of Pediatric Gastroenterology and Nutrition* 2003;36:223-227.

24. Rosenfeldt V, Benfeldt E, Nielsen SD, Michaelsen KF, Jeppesen DL, Valerius NH, Paerregaard A. Effect of probiotic Lactobacillus strains in children with atopic dermatitis. *The Journal of Allergy and Clinical Immunology* 2003;111: 389-395.

25. Rautava S, Kalliomaki M, Isolauri E. Probiotics during pregnancy and breastfeeding might confer immunomodulatory protection against atopic disease in the infant. *The Journal of Allergy and Clinical Immunology* 2002;109:119-121.

26. Kalliomaki M, Salminen S, Arvilommi H, Kero P, Koskinen P, Isolauri E. Probiotics in primary prevention of atopic disease: A randomised placebo-controlled trial. *Lancet* 2001;357:1076-1079.

27. Kalliomaki M, Salminen S, Poussa T, Arvilommi H, Isolauri E. Probiotics and prevention of atopic disease: 4-year follow-up of a randomised placebo-controlled trial. *Lancet* 2003;361:1869-1871.

28. Kaila M, Isolauri E, Soppi E, Virtanen E, Laine S, Arvilommi H. Enhancement of the circulating antibody secreting cell response in human diarrhea by a human Lactobacillus strain. *Pediatric Research* 1992;32:141-144.

29. Gill HS, Rutherfurd KJ, Cross ML, Gopal PK. Enhancement of immunity in the elderly by dietary supplementation with the probiotic *Bifidobacterium lactis* HN019. *American Journal of Clinical Nutrition* 2001;74:833-839.

30. Sheih YH, Chiang BL, Wang LH, Liao CK, Gill HS. Systemic immunity-enhancing effects in healthy subjects following dietary consumption of the lactic acid bacterium *Lactobacillus rhamnosus* HN001. *Journal of the American College of Nutrition* 2001;20:149-156.

31. Wheeler JG, Shema SJ, Bogle ML, Shirrell MA, Burks AW, Pittler A, Helm RM. Immune and clinical impact of *Lactobacillus acidophilus* on asthma. *Annals of Allergy, Asthma and Immunology* 1997;79:229-233.

32. Van de Water J, Keen CL, Gershwin ME. The influence of chronic yogurt consumption on immunity. *The Journal of Nutrition* 1999;129:1492S-1495S.

Chapter 8

1. Kato I, Endo-Tanaka K, Yokokura T. Suppressive effects of the oral administration of *Lactobacillus casei* on type II collagen-induced arthritis in DBA/1 mice. *Life Sciences* 1998;63:635-644.

2. Peltonen R, Nenonen M, Helve T, Hanninen O, Toivanen P, Eerola E. Faecal microbial flora and disease activity in rheumatoid arthritis during a vegan diet. *British Journal of Rheumatology* 1997;36:64-68.

3. Hatakka K, Martio J, Korpela M, Herranen M, Poussa T, Laasanen T, Saxelin M, Vapaatalo H, Moilanen E, Korpela R. Effects of probiotic therapy on the activity and activation of mild rheumatoid arthritis—a pilot study. *Scandinavian Journal of Rheumatology* 2003;32:211-215.

4. McFarland LV. A review of the evidence of health claims for biotherapeutic agents. *Microbial Ecology in Health and Disease* 2000;12:65-76.

5. Salminen S, Bouley C, Boutron-Ruault MC, Cummings JH, Franck A, Gibson GR, Isolauri E, Moreau MC, Roberfroid M, Rowland I. Functional food science and gastrointestinal physiology and function. *The British Journal of Nutrition* 1998;80 Suppl 1:S147-S171.

6. Moore WE, Moore LH. Intestinal floras of populations that have a high risk of colon cancer. *Applied and Environmental Microbiology* 1995;61:3202-3207.

7. Aso Y, Akazan H. Prophylactic effect of a *Lactobacillus casei* preparation on the recurrence of superficial bladder cancer. BLP Study Group. *Urologia Internationalis* 1992;49:125-29.

8. Aso Y, Akaza H, Kotake T, Tsukamoto T, Imai K, Naito S. Preventive effect of a *Lactobacillus casei* preparation on the recurrence of superficial bladder cancer in a double-blind trial. The BLP Study Group. *European Urology* 1995;27:104-109.

9. Okawa T, Niibe H, Arai T, Sekiba K, Noda K, Takeuchi S, Hashimoto S, Ogawa N. Effect of LC9018 combined with radiation therapy on carcinoma of the uterine cervix. A phase III, multicenter, randomized, controlled study. *Cancer* 1993; 72:1949-1954.

10. Okawa T, Kita M, Arai T, Iida K, Dokiya T, Takegawa Y, Hirokawa Y, Yamazaki K, Hashimoto S. Phase II randomized clinical trial of LC9018 concurrently used with radiation in the treatment of carcinoma of the uterine cervix. Its effect on tumor reduction and histology. *Cancer* 1989;64:1769-1776.

11. Agerholm-Larsen L, Bell ML, Grunwald GK, Astrup A. The effect of a probiotic milk product on plasma cholesterol: A meta-analysis of short-term intervention studies. *European Journal of Clinical Nutrition* 2000;54:856-860.

12. Taylor GR, Williams CM. Effects of probiotics and prebiotics on blood lipids. *The British Journal of Nutrition* 1998;80:S225-S230.

13. Anderson JW, Gilliland SE. Effect of fermented milk (yogurt) containing *Lactobacillus acidophilus* L1 on serum cholesterol in hypercholesterolemic humans. *Journal of the American College of Nutrition* 1999;18:43-50.

14. Bertolami MC, Faludi AA, Batlouni M. Evaluation of the effects of a new fermented milk product (Gaio) on primary hypercholesterolemia. *European Journal of Clinical Nutrition* 1999;53:97-101.

15. St Onge MP, Farnworth ER, Savard T, Chabot D, Mafu A, Jones PJ. Kefir consumption does not alter plasma lipid levels or cholesterol fractional synthesis rates relative to milk in hyperlipidemic men: A randomized controlled trial [ISRCTN10820810]. *Biomedical Chromatography Complementary and Alternative Medicine* 2002;2:1.

16. Wang J, Lu Z, Chi J. Multicenter clinical trial of the serum lipid-lowering effects of a *Monascus purpureus* (red yeast) rice preparation from traditional Chinese medicine. *Current Therapeutic Research* 1997;58:964-978.

17. Heber D, Yip I, Ashley JM, Elashoff DA, Elashoff RM, Go VL. Cholesterol-lowering effects of a proprietary Chinese red-yeast-rice dietary supplement. *American Journal of Clinical Nutrition* 1999;69:231-236.

18. Keithley JK, Swanson B, Sha BE, Zeller JM, Kessler HA, Smith KY. A pilot study of the safety and efficacy of cholestin in treating HIV-related dyslipidemia. *Nutrition* 2002;18:201-204.

19. Zhao SP, Liu L, Cheng YC, Li YL. Effect of xuezhikang, a cholestin extract, on reflecting postprandial triglyceridemia after a high-fat meal in patients with coronary heart disease. *Atherosclerosis* 2003;168:375-380.

20. Patrick L, Uzick M. Cardiovascular disease: C-reactive protein and the inflammatory disease paradigm: HMG-CoA reductase inhibitors, alpha-tocopherol, red yeast rice, and olive oil polyphenols. A review of the literature. *Alternative Medicine Review* 2001;6:248-271.

21. Mohan JC, Arora R, Khalilullah M. Preliminary observations on effect of *Lactobacillus sporogenes* on serum lipid levels in hypercholesterolemic patients. *The Indian Journal of Medical Research* 1990;92:431-432.

22. Nase L, Hatakka K, Savilahti E, Saxelin M, Ponka A, Poussa T, Korpela R, Meurman JH. Effect of long-term consumption of a probiotic bacterium, *Lactobacillus rhamnosus* GG, in milk on dental caries and caries risk in children. *Caries Research* 2001;35:412-420.

23. Ahola AJ, Yli-Knuuttila H, Suomalainen T, Poussa T, Ahlstrom A, Meurman JH, Korpela R. Short-term consumption of probiotic-containing cheese and its effect on dental caries risk factors. *Archives of Oral Biology* 2002;47:799-804.

24. Montalto M, Vastola M, Marigo L, Covino M, Graziosetto R, Curigliano V, Santoro L, Cuoco L, Manna R, Gasbarrini G. Probiotic treatment increases salivary counts of lactobacilli: A double-blind, randomized, controlled study. *Digestion* 2004;69:53-56.

25. Voronin AA, Taranenko LA, Sidorenko SV. [Treatment of intestinal dysbacteriosis in children with diabetes mellitus]. *Antibiotiki I Khimioterapii* 1999; 44:22-24.

26. Matsuzaki T, Yamazaki R, Hashimoto S, Yokokura T. Antidiabetic effects of an oral administration of *Lactobacillus casei* in a non-insulin-dependent diabetes mellitus (NIDDM) model using KK-Ay mice. *Endocrine Journal* 1997;44:357-365.

27. Li Z, Yang S, Lin H, Huang J, Watkins PA, Moser AB, Desimone C, Song XY, Diehl AM. Probiotics and antibodies to TNF inhibit inflammatory activity and improve nonalcoholic fatty liver disease. *Hepatology* 2003;37:343-350.

28. Liu Q, Duan ZP, Ha dK, Bengmark S, Kurtovic J, Riordan SM. Synbiotic modulation of gut flora: Effect on minimal hepatic encephalopathy in patients with cirrhosis. *Hepatology* 2004;39:1441-1449.

29. Loguercio C, Abbiati R, Rinaldi M, Romano A, Del Vecchio BC, Coltorti M. Long-term effects of *Enterococcus faecium* SF68 versus lactulose in the treatment of patients with cirrhosis and grade 1-2 hepatic encephalopathy. *Journal of Hepatology* 1995;23:39-46.

30. Read AE, McCarthy CF, Heaton KW, Laidlaw J. *Lactobacillus acidophilus* (enpac) in treatment of hepatic encephalopathy. *British Medical Journal* 1966; 5498:1267-1269.

31. McFarland LV. Do probiotics have a role in the treatment and prevention of nosocomial infections. *Australian Infection Control* 2005;10:12-22.

32. Gluck U, Gebbers JO. Ingested probiotics reduce nasal colonization with pathogenic bacteria (*Staphylococcus aureus*, *Streptococcus pneumoniae*, and beta-hemolytic streptococci). *American Journal of Clinical Nutrition* 2003;77:517-520.

33. Jain PK, McNaught CE, Anderson AD, MacFie J, Mitchell CJ. Influence of synbiotic containing *Lactobacillus acidophilus* La5, *Bifidobacterium lactis* Bb 12, *Streptococcus thermophilus*, *Lactobacillus bulgaricus* and oligofructose on gut barrier function and sepsis in critically ill patients: A randomised controlled trial. *Clinical Nutrition* 2004;23:467-475.

34. Naruszewicz M, Johansson ML, Zapolska-Downar D, Bukowska H. Effect of *Lactobacillus plantarum* 299v on cardiovascular disease risk factors in smokers. *American Journal of Clinical Nutrition* 2002;76:1249-1255.

35. Hata Y, Yamamoto M, Ohni M, Nakajima K, Nakamura Y, Takano T. A placebo-controlled study of the effect of sour milk on blood pressure in hypertensive subjects. *American Journal of Clinical Nutrition* 1996;64:767-771.

36. Gill HS, Rutherfurd KJ, Cross ML, Gopal PK. Enhancement of immunity in the elderly by dietary supplementation with the probiotic *Bifidobacterium lactis* HN019. *American Journal of Clinical Nutrition* 2001;74:833-839.

37. Isolauri E, Sutas Y, Kankaanpaa P, Arvilommi H, Salminen S. Probiotics: Effects on immunity. *American Journal of Clinical Nutrition* 2001;73:444S-450S.

38. Marteau P, Vaerman JP, Dehennin JP, Bord S, Brassart D, Pochart P, Desjeux JF, Rambaud JC. Effects of intrajejunal perfusion and chronic ingestion of *Lactobacillus johnsonii* strain La1 on serum concentrations and jejunal secretions of immunoglobulins and serum proteins in healthy humans. *Gastroentérologie Clinique et Biologique* 1997;21:293-298.

39. Fang H, Elina T, Heikki A, Seppo S. Modulation of humoral immune response through probiotic intake. *Federation of European Microbiological Societies Immunology and Medical Microbiology* 2000;29:47-52.

40. Van de WJ, Keen CL, Gershwin ME. The influence of chronic yogurt consumption on immunity. *The Journal of Nutrition* 1999;129:1492S-1495S.

41. Turchet P, Laurenzano M, Auboiron S, Antoine JM. Effect of fermented milk containing the probiotic *Lactobacillus casei* DN-114001 on winter infections in free-living elderly subjects: A randomised, controlled pilot study. *The Journal of Nutrition, Health and Aging* 2003;7:75-77.

42. Kaila M, Isolauri E, Soppi E, Virtanen E, Laine S, Arvilommi H. Enhancement of the circulating antibody secreting cell response in human diarrhea by a human Lactobacillus strain. *Pediatric Research* 1992;32:141-144.

43. Qamar A, Aboudola S, Warny M, Michetti P, Pothoulakis C, Lamont JT, Kelly CP. *Saccharomyces boulardii* stimulates intestinal immunoglobulin A immune response to *Clostridium difficile* toxin A in mice. *Infection and Immunity* 2001;69:2762-2765.

44. Armuzzi A, Cremonini F, Ojetti V, Bartolozzi F, Canducci F, Candelli M, Santarelli L, Cammarota G, De Lorenzo A, Pola P, et al. Effect of *Lactobacillus* GG supplementation on antibiotic-associated gastrointestinal side effects during *Helicobacter pylori* eradication therapy: A pilot study. *Digestion* 2001;63:1-7.

45. Hamilton-Miller JM. The role of probiotics in the treatment and prevention of *Helicobacter pylori* infection. *International Journal of Antimicrobial Agents* 2003;22:360-366.

46. Wang KY, Li SN, Liu CS, Perng DS, Su YC, Wu DC, Jan CM, Lai CH, Wang TN, Wang WM. Effects of ingesting Lactobacillus- and Bifidobacterium-containing yogurt in subjects with colonized *Helicobacter pylori*. *American Journal of Clinical Nutrition* 2004;80:737-741.

47. Cats A, Kuipers EJ, Bosschaert MA, Pot RG, Vandenbroucke-Grauls CM, Kusters JG. Effect of frequent consumption of a *Lactobacillus casei*-containing milk drink in *Helicobacter pylori*-colonized subjects. *Alimentary Pharmacology and Therapeutics* 2003;17:429-435.

48. Cruchet S, Obregon MC, Salazar G, Diaz E, Gotteland M. Effect of the ingestion of a dietary product containing *Lactobacillus johnsonii* La1 on *Helicobacter pylori* colonization in children. *Nutrition* 2003;19:716-721.

49. Buret AG. How stress induces intestinal hypersensitivity. *American Journal of Pathology*. Jan 2006;168(1):3-5.

50. Yang PC, Jury J, Soderholm JD, Sherman PM, McKay DM, Perdue MH. Chronic psychological stress in rats induces intestinal sensitization to luminal antigens. *American Journal of Pathology.* Jan 2006;168(1):104-114; quiz 363.

51. Lencner AA, Lencner CP, Mikelsaar ME, et al. [The quantitative composition of the intestinal lactoflora before and after space flights of different lengths]. *Nahrung.* 1984;28(6-7):607-613.

52. Bengmark S. Ecological control of the gastrointestinal tract. The role of probiotic flora. *Gut.* Jan 1998;42(1):2-7.

53. Lan PT, Sakamoto M, Benno Y. Effects of two probiotic Lactobacillus strains on jejunal and cecal microbiota of broiler chicken under acute heat stress condition as revealed by molecular analysis of 16S rRNA genes. *Microbiol Immunol.* 2004; 48(12):917-929.

54. Ait-Belgnaoui A, Han W, Lamine F, et al. Lactobacillus farciminis treatment suppresses stress induced visceral hypersensitivity: A possible action through interaction with epithelial cell cytoskeleton contraction. *Gut.* Aug 2006;55(8):1090-1094.

55. Luyer MD, Buurman WA, Hadfoune M, et al. Strain-specific effects of probiotics on gut barrier integrity following hemorrhagic shock. *Infect Immun.* Jun 2005;73(6):3686-3692.

56. Zareie M, Johnson-Henry KC, Jury J, et al. Probiotics prevent bacterial translocation and improve intestinal barrier function in rats following chronic psychological stress. *Gut.* Apr 25 2006.

57. Brudnak MA. Weight-loss drugs and supplements: Are there safer alternatives? *Medical Hypotheses* 2002;58:28-33.

58. St Onge MP. Dietary fats, teas, dairy, and nuts: Potential functional foods for weight control? *American Journal of Clinical Nutrition* 2005;81:7-15.

59. Zemel MB. Regulation of adiposity and obesity risk by dietary calcium: Mechanisms and implications. *Journal of the American College of Nutrition* 2002; 21:146S-151S.

60. Zemel MB, Richards J, Mathis S, Milstead A, Gebhardt L, Silva E. Dairy augmentation of total and central fat loss in obese subjects. *International Journal of Obesity* 2005;29:391-397.

Chapter 11

1. Ishibashi N, Yamazaki S. Probiotics and safety. *American Journal of Clinical Nutrition* 2001;73:465S-470S.

2. Sipsas NV, Zonios DI, Kordossis T. Safety of Lactobacillus strains used as probiotic agents. *Clinical Infectious Diseases* 2002;34:1283-1284.

3. Borriello SP, Hammes WP, Holzapfel W, Marteau P, Schrezenmeir J, Vaara M, Valtonen V. Safety of probiotics that contain lactobacilli or bifidobacteria. *Clinical Infectious Diseases* 2003;36:775-780.

4. Surawicz CM, McFarland LV. Risks of biotherapeutic agents. In: Elmer GW, McFarland LV, Surawicz CM, eds. *Biotherapeutic Agents and Infectious Diseases.* Totowa: Humana Press, 1999:263-268.

5. McFarland LV, Surawicz CM, Greenberg RN, Fekety R, Elmer GW, Moyer KA, Melcher SA, Bowen KE, Cox JL, Noorani Z, et al. Randomized placebo-con-

trolled trial of *Saccharomyces boulardii* in combination with standard antibiotics for *Clostridium difficile* disease. *Journal of American Medical Association* 1994; 271:1913-1918.

6. MacGregor G, Smith AJ, Thakker B, Kinsella J. Yoghurt biotherapy: Contraindicated in immunosuppressed patients? *Postgraduate Medical Journal* 2002;78: 366-367.

7. Rautio M, Jousimies-Somer H, Kauma H, Pietarinen I, Saxelin M, Tynkkynen S, Koskela M. Liver abscess due to a *Lactobacillus rhamnosus* strain indistinguishable from *L. rhamnosus strain* GG. *Clinical Infectious Diseases* 1999;28:1159-1160.

8. Young RJ, Vanderhoof JA. Two cases of Lactobacillus bacteremia during probiotic treatment of short gut syndrome. *Journal of Pediatric Gastroenterology and Nutrition* 2004;39:436-437.

9. Hennequin C, Kauffmann-Lacroix C, Jobert A, Viard JP, Ricour C, Jacquemin JL, Berche P. Possible role of catheters in *Saccharomyces boulardii* fungemia. *European Journal of Clinical Microbiology and Infectious Diseases* 2000;19:16-20.

10. Kniehl E, Becker A, Forster DH. Pseudo-outbreak of toxigenic *Bacillus cereus* isolated from stools of three patients with diarrhoea after oral administration of a probiotic medication. *The Journal of Hospital Infection* 2003;55:33-38.

11. Saxelin M, Chuang NH, Chassy B, Rautelin H, Makela PH, Salminen S, Gorbach SL. Lactobacilli and bacteremia in southern Finland, 1989-1992. *Clinical Infectious Diseases* 1996;22:564-566.

12. Salminen MK, Tynkkynen S, Rautelin H, Saxelin M, Vaara M, Ruutu P, Sarna S, Valtonen V, Jarvinen A. Lactobacillus bacteremia during a rapid increase in probiotic use of *Lactobacillus rhamnosus* GG in Finland. *Clinical Infectious Diseases* 2002;35:1155-1160.

13. Salminen MK, Rautelin H, Tynkkynen S, Poussa T, Saxelin M, Valtonen V, Jarvinen A. Lactobacillus bacteremia, clinical significance, and patient outcome, with special focus on probiotic *L. rhamnosus* GG. *Clinical Infectious Diseases* 2004;38:62-69.

14. McFarland LV. Quality control and regulatory issues for biotherapeutic agents. In: Elmer GW, McFarland LV, Surawicz CM, eds. *Biotherapeutic Agents and Infectious Diseases*. Totowa, NJ: Humana Press, 1999:1-26.

15. Hughes VL, Hillier SL. Microbiologic characteristics of Lactobacillus products used for colonization of the vagina. *Obstetrics and Gynecology* 1990;75:244-248.

16. Clements ML, Levine MM, Ristaino PA, Daya VE, Hughes TP. Exogenous lactobacilli fed to man—their fate and ability to prevent diarrheal disease. *Progress in Food and Nutrition Science* 1983;7:29-37.

17. Green DH, Wakeley PR, Page A, Barnes A, Baccigalupi L, Ricca E, Cutting SM. Characterization of two Bacillus probiotics. *Applied and Environmental Microbiology* 1999;65:4288-4291.

18. Hamilton-Miller JM, Shah S, Smith CT. "Probiotic" remedies are not what they seem. *British Medical Journal* 1996;312:55-56.

19. Hamilton-Miller JM, Shah S, Winkler JT. Public health issues arising from microbiological and labelling quality of foods and supplements containing probiotic microorganisms. *Public Health Nutrition* 1999;2:223-229.

20. Schillinger U. Isolation and identification of lactobacilli from novel-type probiotic and mild yoghurts and their stability during refrigerated storage. *International Journal of Food Microbiology* 1999;47:79-87.

21. Yeung PS, Sanders ME, Kitts CL, Cano R, Tong PS. Species-specific identification of commercial probiotic strains. *Journal of Dairy Science* 2002;85:1039-1051.

22. Zhong W, Millsap K, Bialkowska-Hobrzanska H, Reid G. Differentiation of Lactobacillus species by molecular typing. *Applied and Environmental Microbiology* 1998;64:2418-2423.

23. Canganella F, Paganini S, Ovidi M, Vettraino AM, Bevilacqua L, Massa S, Trovatelli LD. A microbiology investigation on probiotic pharmaceutical products used for human health. *Microbiological Research* 1997;152:171-179.

Index

Page numbers followed by the letter "f" indicate figures; those followed by the letter "t" indicate tables.

Order a copy of this book with this form or online at:
http://www.haworthpress.com/store/product.asp?sku=5597

THE POWER OF PROBIOTICS
Improving Your Health with Beneficial Microbes

_____ in hardbound at $29.95 (ISBN-13: 978-0-7890-2900-3; ISBN-10: 0-7890-2900-6)

_____ in softbound at $19.95 (ISBN-13: 978-0-7890-2901-0; ISBN-10: 0-7890-2901-4)

227 pages plus index • Includes photos and illustrations

Or order online and use special offer code HEC25 in the shopping cart.

COST OF BOOKS_____

☐ **BILL ME LATER:** (Bill-me option is good on US/Canada/Mexico orders only; not good to jobbers, wholesalers, or subscription agencies.)

☐ Check here if billing address is different from shipping address and attach purchase order and billing address information.

POSTAGE & HANDLING_____
(US: $4.00 for first book & $1.50 for each additional book)
(Outside US: $5.00 for first book & $2.00 for each additional book)

Signature_____

SUBTOTAL_____

☐ **PAYMENT ENCLOSED: $**_____

IN CANADA: ADD 6% GST_____

☐ **PLEASE CHARGE TO MY CREDIT CARD.**

STATE TAX_____
(NJ, NY, OH, MN, CA, IL, IN, PA, & SD residents, add appropriate local sales tax)

☐ Visa ☐ MasterCard ☐ AmEx ☐ Discover
☐ Diner's Club ☐ Eurocard ☐ JCB

Account # _____

FINAL TOTAL_____
(If paying in Canadian funds, convert using the current exchange rate, UNESCO coupons welcome)

Exp. Date_____

Signature_____

Prices in US dollars and subject to change without notice.

NAME_____

INSTITUTION_____

ADDRESS_____

CITY_____

STATE/ZIP_____

COUNTRY_____ COUNTY (NY residents only)_____

TEL_____ FAX_____

E-MAIL_____

May we use your e-mail address for confirmations and other types of information? ☐ Yes ☐ No
We appreciate receiving your e-mail address and fax number. Haworth would like to e-mail or fax special discount offers to you, as a preferred customer. **We will never share, rent, or exchange your e-mail address or fax number.** We regard such actions as an invasion of your privacy.

Order From Your Local Bookstore or Directly From
The Haworth Press, Inc.
10 Alice Street, Binghamton, New York 13904-1580 • USA
TELEPHONE: 1-800-HAWORTH (1-800-429-6784) / Outside US/Canada: (607) 722-5857
FAX: 1-800-895-0582 / Outside US/Canada: (607) 771-0012
E-mail to: orders@haworthpress.com

For orders outside US and Canada, you may wish to order through your local
sales representative, distributor, or bookseller.
For information, see http://haworthpress.com/distributors

(Discounts are available for individual orders in US and Canada only, not booksellers/distributors.)
PLEASE PHOTOCOPY THIS FORM FOR YOUR PERSONAL USE.
http://www.HaworthPress.com   BOF07

Dear Customer:

Please fill out & return this form to receive special deals & publishing opportunities for you! These include:
- availability of new books in your local bookstore or online
- one-time prepublication discounts
- free or heavily discounted related titles
- free samples of related Haworth Press periodicals
- publishing opportunities in our periodicals or Book Division

❑ OK! Please keep me on your regular mailing list and/or e-mailing list for new announcements!

Name _____

Address_____

_____

*E-mail address _____
*Your e-mail address will never be rented, shared, exchanged, sold, or divested. You may "opt-out" at any time.
May we use your e-mail address for confirmations and other types of information? ❑ Yes ❑ No

Special
Descri
- For
- Nev
- Pub
- Fr

Spe

_____   _____

_____   _____

_____   _____

Plea   ct:

_____   _____

_____   _____

_____   _____

The

STAPLE OR TAPE YOUR BUSINESS CARD HERE!

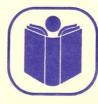
GBIC07